OBSTETRICAL PEARLS

D0596935

OBSTETRICAL PEARLS

THIRD EDITION

MICHAEL D. BENSON, MD, FACOG

Lecturer
Department of Obstetrics and Gynecology
Northwestern University Medical School
Chicago, Illinois

F. A. DAVIS COMPANY • Philadelphia

F. A. Davis Company
1915 Arch Street
Philadelphia, PA 19103

Printed in Canada

Last digit indicates print number: 10 9 8 7 6 5 4 3 2

Acquisitions Editor: Robert W. Reinhardt
Developmental Editor: Bernice M. Wissler
Cover Designer: Louis J. Forgione

As new scientific information becomes available through basic and clinical research, recommended treatments and drug therapies undergo changes. The author(s) and publisher have done everything possible to make this book accurate, up to date, and in accord with accepted standards at the time of publication. The authors, editors, and publisher are not responsible for errors or omissions or for consequences from application of the book, and make no warranty, expressed or implied, in regard to the contents of the book. Any practice described in this book should be applied by the reader in accordance with professional standards of care used in regard to the unique circumstances that may apply in each situation. The reader is advised always to check product information (package inserts) for changes and new information regarding dose and contraindications before administering any drug. Caution is especially urged when using new or infrequently ordered drugs.

Library of Congress Cataloging-in-Publication Data

Benson, Michael D.
    Obstetrical pearls / Michael D. Benson. — 3rd ed.
       p.   cm.
    Includes bibliographical references and index.
    ISBN 0–8036–0432–7
    1. Obstetrics Handbooks, manuals, etc.   2. Pregnancy—
Complications Handbooks, manuals, etc.   I. Title.
    [DNLM: 1. Obstetrics Handbooks.   2. Pregnancy Complications
Handbooks.   WQ 39 B474o 1999]
    RG5391.B46   1999
    618.2—dc21
    DNLM/DLC
    for Library of Congress   99–24043
                                                                    CIP

Foreword

As a medical student or new house officer enters a busy labor and delivery department, it is easy to become overwhelmed. This unique handbook promises to help the obstetrics clerk survive and enjoy his or her obstetrical experience. First, it is more readable than most medical texts and can be entirely digested in about 3 hours. Second, it is designed to emphasize the clinical circumstances faced during the first obstetrics rotation, leaving one to turn to traditional texts for discussion of principles and pathophysiology. Third, it includes an easy approach to situations that are often assumed to be mundane but are described poorly or not at all in other texts. Examples are techniques for obtaining fetal scalp pH, placing a fetal scalp electrode or intrauterine pressure catheter, and performing a circumcision. The approach to obtaining a surgical consent and the proper manner of dictating a concise operative report are clearly detailed. Fourth, this text is cleverly organized by hospital geography rather than by disease, and thereby introduces young physicians to problems that they will face in a given location.

This text is not intended to be a comprehensive treatise on normal or complicated obstetrics. Rather, it is an attempt to facilitate the transition from being a student to being a clinician. As one who has been actively involved in medical student and resident education for the last 20 years, I applaud this novel endeavor as a valuable, efficient teaching aid.

Michael L. Socol, MD
Professor and Vice Chair
Head, Section of Maternal-Fetal Medicine
Department of Obstetrics and Gynecology
Northwestern University Medical School
Chicago, Illinois

Preface

This book was written with some unique objectives in mind:

- To cover 95% of what a medical student through a second-year OB resident is likely to see
- To avoid uncommon conditions, so that 95% of what is in the text is likely to be encountered by the physician in training
- To accomplish these objectives in a text that can be read in its entirety in 3 to 4 hours

When I was in medical school and residency, the standard text was 500 to 1000 pages long, and most of the material covered illnesses that I would never see. The information that I needed on a day-to-day basis was present but distributed throughout the text. The clinical adage, "When you hear hoof beats, think of horses, not zebras," was not followed when it came to the medical education literature—more time was actually spent in describing the rare conditions than the common ones. This text is meant to remedy this deficiency.

Obstetrical Pearls is now in its third edition. The concept has proven successful enough that it has spawned an entire series of "Pearls" books and has been translated into Spanish, Japanese, and Portuguese.

In revising and updating the book, a key concern has been to make it readable and topical. New features have been introduced into this edition: particularly important points are highlighted as "Pearls," and statements about which there is debate or controversy are similarly identified as "Controversies."

As an obstetrician in private practice for over a decade, I am struck by how much change has occurred since the first edition appeared. HIV and hepatitis B were not routinely screened for in obstetrical practice, Beta strep protocols had not been developed, and artificial surfactant for premature infants was found only in the laboratory. Vaginal delivery after a cesarean was still a new concept. Yet the old adage, "The more things change the more they stay the same," remains true today. There is still a need for a compact, easy-to-read text that will allow the physician in training to feel comfortable dealing with the common illnesses and situations that he or she will encounter on a daily basis. I hope that *Obstetrical Pearls* will fill this need.

MDB

Contents

1
PART

Prenatal Care

1
CHAPTER

The Initial Assessment

INITIAL HISTORY

The initial history and physical for obstetrics is similar to that in other rotations. Although it shares features of the labor and delivery history and physical described in a later section, the emphasis is different. Most clinics use a standardized form that is self-explanatory. If not, the history portion can follow the format below.

History of Present Illness

This part of the initial history should focus particularly on prior types of contraception, menstrual history, first positive pregnancy test, and symptoms of pregnancy.

A source of constant confusion is that of gravidity and parity. **PEARL: Gravidity refers to the total number of pregnancies, including the present one. Multiple gestations are counted as only one pregnancy. Parity describes pregnancy outcome. One** method to record parity is to use the T-P-A-L system in which *T* stands for *term,* *P* indicates *preterm deliveries,* *A* refers to *abortions* (whether elective or spontaneous), and *L* is the number of offspring currently *living.* *Full term* in this case means that the fetus was delivered at 37 completed weeks or beyond. In other words, *term* defines a period from 14 days before the due date to 14 days after the due date. An abortion is the intended or unintended delivery of the pregnancy before the fetus completed 20 weeks or achieved 500 g in weight. *Premature* is that time period after 20 weeks and before term.

Past Medical History

Prior abdominal surgery, major medical conditions, and previous pregnancy outcomes are of special interest.

Family History

Predispositions for illness in the mother, such as heart disease or diabetes, are important and include genetic issues for the fetus. Genetic issues refer to birth defects in the families of either parent-to-be, as well as their ethnic backgrounds.

Social History

Substance abuse is of supreme interest here because smoking, alcohol, and drugs can all cause bad outcomes that are presumably preventable. When asking about drug use, phrase the question, "Do you use any recreational drugs such as marijuana or cocaine?" The response is bound to be different than if you say, "You do not use any illegal drugs, do you?" The prospective mother's economic circumstances and living conditions are also relevant.

Review of Systems

Inquire about symptoms characteristic of pregnancy: heartburn, gas, constipation, nausea, breast tenderness, and the like.

INITIAL PHYSICAL EXAM

The physical exam should include all major body systems, with particular emphasis on the abdomen and pelvis. Scars, presence of heart tones, and uterine size should be included in the abdominal exam. For the pelvic exam, cervical dilatation and effacement as well as uterine size are of interest. Pelvimetry, or estimation of the size of the bony pelvis, is particularly difficult for beginners, but an effort can be made to note some of the most obvious landmarks, which are indicated below and in Figure 1–1.

CONTROVERSY: The utility of pelvimetry is debated because it is not highly reproducible among examiners, and it has not been found to be very accurate in predicting the length or course of labor.

Conjugate Diameter

Conjugate diameter is defined as the distance from the lower aspect of the pubic symphysis to the sacral promontory. To measure this distance,

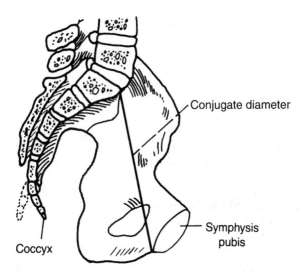

Figure 1-1. The maternal pelvis. (Adapted from Bonica, JJ: Principles and Practice of Obstetric Analgesia and Anesthesia. FA Davis, Philadelphia, 1967, p 851, with permission.)

simply palpate as far upward and backward as possible. Unless you have long fingers, you often will not be able to feel the sacral promontory. In this event, simply note that the CD is greater than the measured length of your outstretched fingers.

Sacrum

Is it hollow or flat? This is a subjective assessment.

Coccyx

Is it anterior or posterior? Again, a matter of judgment.

Ischial Spines

These are the bony protuberances at 4 o'clock and 8 o'clock, 2 inches or so into the vaginal canal along the vaginal sidewalls. Are they prominent?

Transverse Diameter

Transverse diameter is the distance between the ischial tuberosities and can best be examined with the patient flat with her legs adducted and dorsi-flexed (the position for a routine pelvic exam). They are the broad bony prominences that are palpable on the medial aspect of the buttocks, inferior to the anus.

Pubic Arch Angle

The pubic arch angle can be estimated by sweeping two fingers under the pubic arch. Women commonly have an arch angle of 110° or greater.

Pelvimetry is of limited importance in the prenatal evaluation because in most cases, cephalopelvic disproportion (fetus too large for the pelvis) is empirically determined by observing the course of labor.

DATING THE PREGNANCY

Dating the pregnancy is one of the most important tasks in prenatal care.

Last Menstrual Period

It is often stated that 40% of women do not accurately recall their last menstrual period (LMP).

The following facts need to be stated in the chart at the first visit:

1. First day of last menstrual period and whether or not it was normal.
2. The length and variability of the patient's menstrual cycles (when not on oral contraceptives).
3. Presence or absence of pill use or breast-feeding within 6 months prior to conception. These factors can result in delayed ovulation for several subsequent cycles.

First Fetal Movement (Quickening)

Primigravidas generally feel the first fetal movement at 18 to 20 weeks, whereas women with their second pregnancy and beyond feel the fetus move 2 weeks earlier.

Fetal Heartbeat

The heart can be heard with the fetoscope as early as 17 weeks and usually by 20 weeks. The heartbeat can usually be heard with a Doppler instrument by 12 weeks. From 16 weeks and beyond, it is important to document how the heart tones were detected. In this time period, listening with the fetoscope and noting the first date on which the heartbeat can be heard can help confirm the due date. **PEARL: In the first two trimesters, the fetal heartbeat is most commonly heard close to the midline.**

Fundal Height

Measure from the top of the symphysis pubis.

12 weeks: Palpable abdominally just at the symphysis pubis.

16 weeks: Palpable midway between the symphysis and the umbilicus.

20 weeks: Palpable at the umbilicus.

20 to 32 weeks: Height in centimeters above symphysis parallels gestational age in weeks.

Although these guidelines can serve as a rule of thumb, interobserver and intraobserver variability is very high. Assuming that one ultrasound has been previously done to confirm the due date, additional scans based on discrepancies in the physical exam are warranted only in the more extreme cases.

Ultrasound

1. **First trimester:** Crown-rump length predicts the estimated date of confinement (EDC, or due date) to within 7 to 10 days.

2. **Second trimester:** Biparietal diameter (BPD) or femur length predicts EDC to within 7 to 10 days.

3. **Third trimester:** Scans postponed to this time period are not very helpful in predicting the EDC and are accurate only to within 3 weeks either way.

As a rule, when an early ultrasound prediction disagrees with an EDC assigned by the LMP by more than 1 week, the ultrasound dates are assigned. If the scan and the LMP agree to within a week, the EDC based on the LMP is used. This may not always be straightforward because femur length may or may not agree with the estimated gestational age based on the biparietal diameter. **PEARL: Ultrasound is not the last word on dating a pregnancy and must be used in combination with other observations.**

If there is any question concerning the due date assigned on the basis of LMP, an ultrasound should be considered to help clarify the issue. Most patients presenting after 18 weeks should probably be scanned at least once. They should also be scanned if there is a large discrepancy between dates and size or if the uterus does not seem to be growing on several successive visits.

REFERRAL TO A HIGH-RISK CLINIC

Many residency programs have more than one obstetrical clinic or make consultation available for so-called high-risk patients. The following are examples of problems that warrant referral to the high-risk clinic or consultation (when available) for follow-up on future visits:

1. History of preterm delivery (<36 weeks or weight <5 pounds, 8 ounces).
2. Prior intrauterine fetal demise.
3. Pregnancy loss between 14 and 20 weeks (suggestive of incompetent cervix).
4. Multiple gestation.
5. Third-trimester bleeding or the discovery of placenta previa after 26 to 28 weeks' gestation.
6. Isoimmunization.
7. Presence of serious systemic disease, such as diabetes, hypertension, asthma, renal or cardiac disease, etc.
8. History of deep venous thrombosis (not varicose veins) or pulmonary embolus.

2
CHAPTER

Routine Prenatal Visits

Patients are seen monthly until 28 weeks and then every 2 weeks. After 36 weeks, patients are seen weekly. The following items are checked with every prenatal visit.

WEIGHT

Ideally, a patient should gain about 25 to 35 pounds during her pregnancy—roughly ½ pound per week for the first 28 weeks and 1 pound per week thereafter. Many gravidas will not stick closely to this pattern. Obese patients may gain substantially less. Mothers who are gaining too much weight should be encouraged to avoid snacks, watch their consumption of high-calorie fluids (soft drinks, even juices and milk), and stick to three well-balanced meals per day. Weight gain of more than 5 pounds per week at the end of pregnancy may be a sign of pregnancy-induced hypertension, and the urine and blood pressure should be checked closely. Those with extremes of weight gain should have their eating habits reviewed and should be referred to a dietitian if one is available. Weight loss that occurs over more than one visit is of particular concern.

Patients often ask about the safety of artificial sweeteners such as aspartame (NutraSweet). **PEARL: A modified amino acid, aspartame is not a known or suspected teratogen or mutagen, and it has been in the food supply for several decades.** Even for mothers carrying a fetus with phenylketonuria, the additive is safe, as the mother's enzymes break it down; carriers of phenylketonuria are also able to do so. In a real sense, aspartame is safer than sugar, since chronic exposure to large doses of sugar may lead to obesity and an increased risk of cesarean section and diabetes.

BLOOD PRESSURE

The maternal blood pressure tends to drop in the second trimester and rise in the third trimester.

Guidelines for Concern

1. Diastolic greater than 90
2. Systolic of 140 or greater

Work-up

1. Repeat blood pressure both sitting up and in lateral decubitus (upper arm).
2. 24-hour urine for total protein and creatinine clearance.
3. Blood chemistries including creatinine and liver function tests. If the patient is in the third tri-

mester, also CBC with platelets to evaluate for pregnancy-induced hypertension.
4. Stat urinalysis if dipstick urine indicates more than 1+ protein on a voided specimen. A clean-catch midstream or even a catheterized specimen should be obtained if the patient has heavy vaginal discharge.

Follow-up

If elevated blood pressures are recorded at the time of the first visit in the first or early second trimester, they may indicate that the patient is a chronic hypertensive (see Chapter 16).

If these pressures are newly elevated and recorded in the late second trimester or third trimester, the patient may well have pregnancy-induced hypertension. An experienced resident should be notified, because the patient may need to be hospitalized for observation. At the very least, she should be rechecked in 2 to 3 days, and a non-stress test (NST—see Fetal Movement in Chapter 4) may be appropriate (depending on the gestational age and the absolute value of the blood pressure).

URINE DIPSTICK

Protein

A negative, trace, or 1+ reading requires no action. A 2+ or greater reading requires a clean-catch midstream urinalysis (hold for culture and sensitivity). If it is suggestive of a urinary tract infection, the patient may be treated presumptively. She should call 2 or 3 days later for the culture results. The blood pressure must be checked to be sure that it is not elevated. **PEARL: Proteinuria can be a sign of pregnancy-induced hypertension, particularly if accompanied by elevated blood pressure.**

Glucose

Although the threshold for glucosuria in pregnancy is reduced, in practice, glucose is usually absent or weakly positive on dipstick testing. If 2+ glucose is found on a urine dipstick, it may be appropriate to perform the routine diabetes screen earlier than the usual 24 to 28 weeks (see Blood Sugar and Diabetes in Chapter 3). If a screen has already been done, and glucosuria is a repeated finding in the third trimester, there may be merit in rechecking the screening test or even obtaining a more definitive 3-hour glucose tolerance test, although glucosuria is not very specific for gestational diabetes.

FUNDAL HEIGHT
AND FETAL HEARTBEAT

See Dating the Pregnancy in Chapter 1.

EDEMA

PEARL: Reports of edema have ultimately come from 75% of pregnant women. Thus, it is no longer considered a screening sign or symptom for pregnancy-induced hypertension. Those with excessive or sudden swelling should, of course, have their blood pressure and urine protein checked, but usually the swelling is an isolated finding. A good clue to excessive swelling is a weight gain of 3 pounds or more in a week.

Sitting with legs up or lying on one's side will help isolated edema. To be effective, the patient has to rest for several hours when she would not otherwise. In practice, most patients prefer to tolerate moderate leg swelling rather than lie in bed for several hours during the middle of the day.

FETAL MOVEMENT

Fetal movement should be noted on each visit. The first perception by the patient (quickening) should also be noted. Specific instructions for the third trimester are reviewed under Fetal Movement in Chapter 4.

3
CHAPTER

Prenatal Labs

BLOOD SUGAR AND DIABETES

Several hormones of pregnancy are insulin antag-
onists. Chief among them is human placental lac-
togen (HPL), which is secreted by the placenta in
rough proportion to its weight. Thus, women who
have normal glucose tolerances in early pregnancy may actually be diabetic later in the gestation. Prior to the introduction of insulin, 50% of
diabetic mothers died, and the fetal outcome was
worse. This disease is important because it is reasonably common (1% to 2% of pregnant mothers)
and because we can have a significant impact on
its outcome.

Risk Factors

The following features of a patient's initial assessment suggest that the patient is at higher than
average risk for diabetes.

1. Prior stillbirth
2. Prior fetus weighing over 9 pounds
3. Strong family history of diabetes

4. Morbid obesity
5. Glucosuria

Screening Policy

1. All pregnancies should be screened between 24 and 28 weeks with a 1-hour postprandial glucose test. This is a blood test drawn 1 hour after the patient consumes a 50-g glucose load. Many institutions do this after an overnight fast, but others simply administer the glucose during the regular appointment anytime during the day.
2. Those with an abnormal 1-hour postprandial glucose level should have the 3-hour glucose tolerance test as soon as possible. If the result of the test is abnormal, the patient is referred immediately to the diabetic or high-risk clinic.
3. Patients at high risk for gestational diabetes by history might benefit from a glucose screen at presentation or a second screening test at 32 weeks.

The 1-Hour Postprandial Glucose

The patient can be given a 50-g oral glucose load regardless of when she last ate and have her glucose checked 1 hour later. A fasting (or pretest) glucose is not measured with this screen. The cut-off value varies among institutions, but it is usually considered abnormal if it is higher than 140 (mg/100 mL). **PEARL: About 15% of the population will have an abnormal 1-hour test with this cut-off.**

CONTROVERSY: Some advocate the use of a lower cut-off of 130, which would increase the sensitivity of the test but subject 25% of the population to additional testing.

The 3-Hour Glucose Tolerance Test

The patient is to have 100-g carbohydrate intake for 3 days prior to the test. The test requires administration of a 100-g glucose load and then checking the plasma glucose at fasting, 1 hour, 2 hours, and 3 hours. The upper limit of normal for each of the values (plasma in mg/100 mL) is

Fasting: 105
1 Hour: 190
2 Hours: 165
3 Hours: 145

The test is abnormal if two or more values exceed the upper limit of normal.

***CONTROVERSY:** A somewhat less popular alternative set of normal values that is used at some institutions is 95 (fasting), 180 (1 hour), 155 (2 hours), and 140 (3 hours).*

Classifying Diabetes

A gestational diabetic is one whose 3-hour glucose tolerance test is abnormal and who was not known to be diabetic prior to the pregnancy. This definition is known to encompass a very heterogeneous group and may include those who should have been on insulin before the pregnancy. (Most women are screened for the first time during pregnancy.) One commonly used classification scheme for describing diabetes in pregnant women (based on the White system) is described in the following list:

Class A-1: Fasting glucose less than 105.
Class A-2: Fasting glucose greater than 105—these patients are usually started on insulin.
Class B-1: Fasting glucose 130 or more.
Class B-2: Adult onset (type II) diabetics (on insulin prior to pregnancy).

Class C: Diabetes onset between ages 10 and 19.
Class D: Diabetes of more than 20 years' duration or beginning before age 10.
Class F: Concomitant nephropathy.
Class R: Malignant retinopathy.
Class H: Heart impairment or disease

Diabetes of any degree establishes a pregnancy as high risk and requires consultation of more senior residents or faculty members.

Problems Faced by Pregnant Diabetics

Diabetics face three special types of difficulties during pregnancy. The risk of congenital malformation, particularly in the heart and nervous system, is greatly increased (especially in those with abnormal glucose tolerance in the first trimester). Generally, these patients have a twofold to fourfold increase in risk, which tends to be higher in those under poor control. The risk of intrauterine fetal demise (stillbirth) is also increased, although this is more of an issue for those requiring insulin prior to pregnancy. Finally, macrosomia, in which the fetus attains an excessive size, is of concern because this condition predisposes to shoulder dystocia and cephalopelvic disproportion. For these reasons, many authorities initiate nonstress tests (NSTs—see Fetal Movement in Chapter 4) in the third trimester and obtain periodic ultrasounds to help identify either macrosomia or placental insufficiency, particularly in insulin-dependent diabetic patients. An experienced obstetrician should be present at the delivery of a diabetic, because shoulder dystocia can be a serious problem. There is substantial debate about the degree of risk for both intrauterine fetal demise and macrosomia in women who develop gestational diabetes.

Because about half of gestational diabetics will

have abnormal glucose tolerance later in life, the American Diabetes Association recommends follow-up testing at their first postpartum visit. The suggested screen is a fasting 75-g, 2-hour glucose tolerance test. Normal values are less than 115 for the fasting sample, less than 200 at 1 hour, and less than 140 at 2 hours. Those with a normal screen should have fasting glucose measurements obtained yearly, with additional testing for values above 115.

HEMATOCRIT

A CBC with red cell indices is typically performed during the first or early second trimester. Hematocrits are routinely rechecked at 24 to 28 weeks, with glucose screening. **PEARL: Because plasma expansion exceeds the proportion of hemoglobin mass increase, the Centers for Disease Control and Prevention have defined anemia as less than 11 g/dL in the first and third trimesters and less than 10.5 g/dL in the second trimester.** A hemoglobin electrophoresis should be obtained in those patients who

1. Are not anemic but have microcytosis (MCV < 80) or hypochromia (MCH < 27)
2. Are anemic but do not have iron deficiency anemia on the basis of low iron, serum ferritin, or transferrin saturation.
3. Appear to have iron deficiency anemia but who do not improve with iron treatment.

A purely iron deficiency anemia will usually respond to iron supplementation within 2 weeks.

Since hemoglobinopathies tend to occur more in specific ethnic groups, prenatal screening should include a hemoglobin electrophoresis for all those with African ancestry. A so-called sickle cell screening test is no longer believed to be sensitive enough to detect all hemoglobin variants. Those with Asian or Mediterranean backgrounds should be asked specifically about anemia and thalassemia; the threshold for obtaining a hemoglobin electrophoresis should be lower for these groups as well.

The partners of pregnant women who have hemoglobin variants demonstrated by testing should also be checked. If both have abnormalities, they should be sent for specialized genetic counseling. **PEARL: Although the couple may not share the same recessive gene, significant disease can arise in offspring who inherit two different hemoglobinopathy traits.** Many hemoglobin abnormalities in the fetus can be detected prenatally through the use of amniocentesis or chorionic villus sampling (CVS) (see Genetic Testing later in this chapter). Women with sickle cell trait are more prone to bacteriuria and therefore pyelonephritis, and should be screened frequently (perhaps monthly) with urine cultures.

Rh AND ANTIBODY SCREEN

Rh-negative mothers receive a passive immunization at 28 weeks to prevent hemolytic disease of the newborn. Without the vaccine before and after birth, Rh-negative mothers may develop antibodies to the Rh antigen if their fetus is Rh-positive. In future pregnancies, these IgG antibodies can cross the placenta and destroy Rh-positive fetal red blood cells. This may lead to severe anemia and death for subsequent Rh-positive fetuses. Although most maternal Rh immunization takes place at the time of birth with the entrance of fetal red blood cells into the bloodstream, a small percentage of pregnant women will be exposed to fetal red blood cells before labor and thus become immunized.

The immunization consists of an injection at 28 weeks with IgG antibody to the Rh antigen. One common brand name of this vaccine is RhoGAM. **PEARL: If an antibody screen is done within weeks (or even 2 to 3 months) after this injection, it may be positive. PEARL: These mothers also must receive RhoGAM for amniocentesis or any other event that places them at increased risk for fetal-maternal transfusion (such as an abortion).** The mothers also receive RhoGAM in the first 3 days postpartum if their child is indeed Rh-positive. It must be remembered that an antibody screen must always be checked prior to giving RhoGAM at any time, to be sure that Rh sensitization has not already taken place.

All positive antibody screens require consultation.

RUBELLA TITER

Most cases of rubella (German measles) are subclinical, so the history is completely unreliable. The rubella virus is a teratogen capable of causing cardiac defects, cataracts, and deafness in the fetus. Nonimmune women should be vaccinated postpartum, as all vaccines use an attenuated live strain of virus and are theoretically teratogenic in and of themselves, although this has not been the case in actual practice. All patients are routinely screened for immunity, and those with borderline values should have the test repeated to be sure that they do not have a current infection.

Those who are vaccinated should avoid pregnancy for 3 months. They are not contagious. The vaccination does not prohibit breast-feeding.

HUMAN IMMUNODEFICIENCY VIRUS (HIV)

Several organizations, including the American College of Obstetricians and Gynecologists and the Centers for Disease Control and Prevention, recommend universal, voluntary screening of pregnant women for HIV infection. The voluntary nature of this screening implies a formal consent process in which patients are advised about the benefits and limitations of testing, the voluntary nature of the test, and the mechanism by which positive results will be disclosed and to whom.

The tests used for screening are enzyme-linked immunosorbent assays (ELISAs) for HIV antibodies. These assays have small but meaningful false-positive and false-negative rates. For instance, it takes several months after infection for most people to develop detectable antibodies. **PEARL: Positive screening tests for HIV must be confirmed by further testing, although protocols vary.** Follow-up testing can include

1. Repeat ELISA test for HIV antibody
2. Western blot test (assay for HIV core and envelope antigens)
3. ELISA test for HIV antigen (AKA p24 antigen test)
4. Tissue culture for virus
5. HIV DNA polymerase chain test

The risk of vertical transmission of this infection (from mother to fetus) can range from 20% to 30% in HIV-positive women. **PEARL: Recent evidence has shown that the HIV transmission rate can be reduced by almost 75% with the antiretroviral agent zidovudine.** The US Public Health Service recommends initiating treatment at 14 to 34 weeks with 100 mg orally five times daily, adding intravenous dosing during labor (2 mg/kg loading dose, followed by 1 mg/kg infusion). This protocol also calls for the treatment of newborns with zidovudine syrup for the first 6 weeks of life. Pregnancy alone is not thought to affect the disease course for the HIV-positive woman.

HEPATITIS B

The rationale for screening pregnant women for hepatitis B is similar to that for HIV—vertical transmission of the infection can be prevented. Typically, screening is performed by testing for hepatitis B surface antigen. If this test is positive, additional serology should be obtained to help define disease status and transmission risk:

- Hepatitis B surface antibody
- Hepatitis B core antigen and antibody
- Hepatitis B e antigen and antibody

Women with both surface and e antigens are at greatest risk for vertical transmission, with estimates ranging as high as 90%. Evidence suggests that infection is most likely to take place during birth or in the first few weeks of life. **PEARL: Current practice is to passively immunize newborns exposed to hepatitis B with immune globulin and to initiate active immunization by starting the vaccination series within the first few days of life.** This approach has been shown to be highly effective in reducing the risk of neonatal infection (to less than 10%).

PAP SMEAR

Pap smear abnormalities can be of two types: those suggesting the presence of an infectious disease and those indicating dysplasia. Infectious diseases identified on a Pap smear (yeast, tricho-monas, etc.) do not need to be treated if the patient is asymptomatic.

Pap smears that are frankly abnormal are classified as a low-grade or high-grade *squamous intraepithelial lesion.* The low-grade lesions may be categorized as condyloma and mild dysplasia, and the high-grade lesions as moderate or severe dysplasia (including carcinoma in situ). With the high-grade lesions, an examination with a colposcope (a type of magnifying glass) and directed biopsies of the cervix are performed in order to exclude malignancy and determine frequency of follow-up.

CONTROVERSY: The proper follow-up of low-grade lesions is controversial, particularly during pregnancy. An alternative to colposcopy and biopsy may be simply follow-up Pap smears at intervals of 3 to 6 months, although the recommendation has to be individualized according to the patient's medical history and likelihood of compliance.

Treatment, such as freezing or lasering of the cervix, is usually postponed to the postpartum period if the lesion is not invasive cancer.

The Pap smear can occasionally be normal in the presence of cancer. Cervices that appear to be very abnormal or that have fungating, indurated regions should be brought to the attention of an experienced examiner. **PEARL: More often than not, the cervix is actually normal, but keep in mind that a normal Pap smear does not absolutely exclude cancer.**

MATERNAL SERUM ALPHA-FETOPROTEIN

This serum test, performed between 15 and 20 weeks of gestation, is used to screen for fetuses with neural tube defects. This group of congenital anomalies occurs at the rate of roughly 1 in 1000 pregnancies (5 in 1000 in the British Isles) and includes a variety of conditions such as spina bifida and anencephaly (fetus missing cerebral cortex). High levels of a specific protein, alpha-fetoprotein (AFP), in the maternal bloodstream may suggest an afflicted fetus.

In the past few years, the test's predictive value has been improved by adding a concomitant assay for HCG, estradiol, or both. This improved test is also known as *the AFP plus test* or the *triple screen*. The addition of a second or even third protein assay makes interpretation of the test significantly more complicated. In many labs, a narrative report accompanies the interpretation. In the case of abnormal values, the lab will typically recommend a specific follow-up (i.e., a repeat test, ultrasound, or amniocentesis). Abnormal values are to be called to the attention of an experienced resident. (Most institutions have a standard protocol about the follow-up of these tests.) With most screening procedures, about 30 to 50 mothers out of 1000 will have an initial abnormal AFP (against a background incidence of 1 to 2 per 1000 with an actual defect). Those morally opposed to abortion may decline this test. **PEARL: Abnormally high AFP levels can occur from incorrect gestational age assignment, twins, and fetal demise.**

Women with one abnormal test (generally 2.5 multiples of the median or higher) should have an ultrasound to confirm the gestational age and rule out twins. If the scan disagrees by more than 7 days with the age assigned by the last menstrual period, the gestational age is changed and the result reinterpreted. If the value remains abnormal, the patient undergoes a combination of genetic counseling and then amniocentesis and an ultrasound to look for anomalies (if she agrees).

Unusually low values (0.5 multiples of the median or less) may predict an increased risk of chromosomal abnormalities (such as Down syndrome).

PEARL: The follow-up of a low AFP differs from that of a high value in that the test is generally not repeated. If the follow-up ultrasound confirms the EDC and provides no other explanation for the low value, genetic counseling and amniocentesis should be offered.

CONTROVERSY: A question that has arisen in recent years is the necessity of an amniocentesis if the second trimester ultrasound is perfectly normal.

In any case, the protocol for following up an abnormal initial test varies among institutions. Whatever method is used, it is important to recognize that the normal range is highly dependent on gestational age and that unusually high or low levels of AFP need to be pursued.

ULTRASOUND

The availability of ultrasound examination and protocols for routine scanning vary greatly among institutions. Nevertheless, once an ultrasound is obtained, the following is a partial list of findings that require consultation:

1. High risk for intrauterine growth retardation (IUGR).
2. Macrosomia (unusually large fetus).
3. Oligohydramnios (abnormally low volume of amniotic fluid).
4. Hydramnios (abnormally high volume of amniotic fluid).
5. Breech presentation or transverse lie after 35 weeks (no need for action before this time).
6. Placenta previa (after 28 weeks—sooner if bleeding).

GENETIC TESTING

Two prenatal tests are available that can identify fetuses with chromosome errors and some specific genetic anomalies: amniocentesis and CVS. The field is advancing so rapidly that any statements committed to print quickly become obsolete. Even so, a few brief principles are worth reviewing.

Amniocentesis

The gold standard of genetic testing, amniocentesis has traditionally been done between 14 to 18 weeks—a time when enough fluid has accumulated to make the test easy to perform but early enough so that if the results are abnormal, the patient can undergo a pregnancy termination. The most common reason for doing the test is to study the fetal chromosomes.

Although there are several different classes of congenital anomalies, chromosome errors are the only type of defect to increase in frequency with advancing maternal age. Since these defects are often severe or even lethal (one example is Down syndrome), it has become common practice to offer prenatal diagnosis for chromosome errors to women who will be 35 years old or older at the time of delivery. This is the first age at which the probability of finding a chromosome error (roughly 1 in 170) exceeds the risk of spontaneous abortion from the procedure itself (1 in 200). It is helpful to realize that most pregnancy losses after the procedure would have occurred anyway. Specifically, 6 in 200 pregnancies viable at 16 weeks are subsequently lost. This number rises only to 7 in 200 after amniocentesis.

The technique relies on the fact that fetal cells shed into the amniotic fluid are still viable and can be cultured to build up enough volume of cells for analysis. Because the cells have to multiply before testing can be performed, it usually takes 2 to 3 weeks to have a karyotype (chromosome count) from the amniotic fluid.

With the advances in biotechnology, an ever-lengthening list of specific genetic errors can also be identified, such as Tay-Sachs disease and, recently, sickle cell anemia. However, amniocentesis is not appropriate for all mothers, and not all tests available can be performed on each fluid sample. Rather, the initial history is used to identify people at increased risk for one or more genetic problems. The most obvious risk is mothers who will be age 35 or older at the time of delivery, but certain ethnic groups might also benefit from genetic screening and, occasionally, amniocentesis. For example, if both members of a Jewish couple are carrying the Tay-Sachs gene, a genetic amniocentesis can identify prenatally those 25% of babies who will have the fatal homozygous disease.

Chorionic Villus Sampling

CVS is a relatively new technique that involves aspirating a very small portion of the placenta at 10 to 12 weeks. The placenta has the fetal karyotype rather than the maternal one. The actual aspiration is performed with ultrasound guidance and can be done either transvaginally or transabdominally. CVS can be done 5 to 6 weeks earlier than amniocentesis, and the results can usually be obtained within a week, since a greater number of fetal cells are obtained from the outset with this technique. CVS can be used both for karyotypes and identifying specific genetic errors, but it cannot yet be used to screen for neural tube defects because this requires measurement of amniotic fluid AFP. Rarely, a patient who undergoes CVS will have an elevated serum AFP and require amniocentesis.

The compelling advantage of CVS is that results can be obtained in the first trimester rather than the second trimester as with amniocentesis. This is of great practical importance for those who wish to terminate an abnormal pregnancy.

CONTROVERSY: The disadvantage of CVS is its slightly higher loss rate (on the order of 1 to 2 per 200) when compared with the 1 per 200 of amniocentesis, although (as with amniocentesis) most losses after CVS would have occurred anyway. Another issue that has arisen regarding the safety of CVS involves the potential increased risk of a specific birth defect known as limb reduction anomalies. Estimates of the risk of a defect involving the limbs or digits vary widely, but a commonly accepted number is that the risk is on the order of 1 in 3000.

4
CHAPTER

Common Concerns and Problems of Pregnant Women

FETAL MOVEMENT

If a patient complains of decreased fetal movement after 28 weeks, she needs a nonstress test (NST) that day. An NST should not be ordered weekly thereafter for this nonrecurring problem.

The NST consists of electronically monitoring and recording the fetal pulse rate for a minimum of 20 minutes. A *reactive* NST is one that is reassuring about fetal well-being. While the definition of *reactive* varies among institutions, a common one is a pulse pattern with two or more accelerations lasting for at least 15 seconds within a 20-minute period, with the peak of the acceleration being 15 BPM above the baseline fetal heart rate (FHR). The interpretation of FHR tracings is described in greater detail in Fetal Monitoring in Chapter 6.

With regard to monitoring fetal movement in general, there are a variety of different protocols for instructing patients. An example of one such guideline is as follows:

1. Upon awakening, begin counting your baby's movements.
2. A kick, punch, or roll each counts as one movement. If the baby kicks and then rolls, this should be counted as two movements.
3. Stop counting for the day when you reach 10. The baby is fine.
4. If you don't reach 10 by 5 PM, call your doctor. You will need to come in for an NST (the nurse will place a monitor on your abdomen for half an hour to hear the baby's pulse). Most babies are just fine.

The key principle is that any large change in the fetal daily activity requires follow-up.

CONTROVERSY: In some studies, the stillbirth rate has been shown to decrease significantly among mothers who monitor their baby's movements daily.

VAGINAL INFECTIONS

Single women should probably be checked for gonorrhea and chlamydia during their first prenatal visit. Erythromycin should be used for treatment instead of tetracycline, which potentially may discolor fetal teeth. Symptomatic yeast infections can be treated with either over-the-counter medication or prescription creams and suppositories. Metronidazole (Flagyl) can be given during pregnancy, but the manufacturer recommends withholding it during the first trimester, because it is known to cross the placenta.

URINARY TRACT INFECTIONS

Treat urinary tract infections as you would normally. Pregnant women may be more prone to urinary tract infections, and some institutions routinely obtain cultures to detect asymptomatic bacteriuria. **PEARL: Once an infection is established, a culture should be obtained following treatment and periodically thereafter, perhaps monthly.** Never prescribe tetracycline during pregnancy, and avoid, if possible, giving sulfa or nitrofurantoin after 36 weeks. Tetracycline administered during pregnancy can cause permanent discoloration of the offspring's teeth. Sulfa drugs administered close to the time of delivery can presumably displace bilirubin from its carrier molecules and theoretically can predispose to kernicterus, a condition with severe neural symptoms. Nitrofurantoin might exacerbate hemolytic anemias resulting from immature erythrocyte enzymes in the fetus, and therefore the drug should not be given to pregnant women at term.

SEX

There are no restrictions placed on sex for the pregnant woman without specific medical or obstetrical problems. Air emboli resulting in maternal death have been reported in the medical literature from blowing air under pressure into the vagina during oral sex.

ABDOMINAL PAIN

Most pregnant women eventually complain of lower abdominal discomfort or pain. Sometimes the pain may actually be a uterine contraction. **PEARL: Patients at 24 weeks and beyond should be advised to call if they have frequent contractions (greater than four per hour) for 2 consecutive hours, because this may be an early sign of preterm labor.** This discomfort may actually be Braxton Hicks contractions (isolated, generally mild tightening sensations of the uterus), but often it is hard to find a specific cause. Occasionally, patients will be tender along the lateral aspects of the uterus. This condition is commonly referred to as *round ligament pain* because it corresponds roughly to the location of the round ligament, although the physiology behind the pain is poorly delineated. Mild abdominal aches and pains can be treated with a heating pad and acetaminophen (Tylenol).

LEG CRAMPS

Many pregnant women experience painful leg cramping, particularly at night. The cause of these cramps is unknown. Although uncomfortable, most patients are satisfied with reassurance that this is a normal discomfort of pregnancy. For those with particularly bad symptoms, supplemental calcium can be tried (although the evidence of benefit is skimpy at best). Physical examination should be performed at some point, however, to rule out deep venous thrombosis. If the physical exam is suspicious (such as demonstrating asymmetric swelling, localized tenderness, cords, or erythema), duplex imaging should be ordered, because examination by itself is notoriously unreliable. Duplex imaging consists of a real-time ultrasound study of the venous circulation between the knee and the groin. Deep venous thromboses can actually be visualized with this technique.

COMMON MYTHS

- **NutraSweet is not safe during pregnancy.** The sweetener is safe for all except women known to be homozygous for phenylketonuria. NutraSweet is a combination of two amino acids, phenylalanine and aspartic acid.
- **The fetal heart rate is linked to gender.** The heart rate varies from instant to instant, so this idea falls apart under the briefest scrutiny.
- **Women are more likely to go into labor during a full moon.** Scientifically studied, this is simply not true.
- **Pregnant women are more likely to rupture membranes before storms.** Although it is true that atmospheric pressure drops with rain, so does the pressure within the body, which is equal at all times with the external pressure. If it were not, more than the amnionic membranes would burst.
- **Pregnant women should not sleep on their backs.** A particularly persistent myth, its origins can probably be traced to the observation that labor in the supine position can compromise uterine blood flow. This is not relevant to nonlaboring patients (and not terribly important for those in labor). Although many women are uncomfortable flat on their back and can even develop symptomatic hypotension, those who can tolerate this position will not cause fetal injury. (Those who cannot will simply avoid the position naturally.)
- **Hot baths can injure the fetus.** Although some data do link increases in maternal core temperatures with birth defects, it is nearly impossible to raise core temperature from a hot bath. Total body immersion in warm water may raise body temperature, but as a practical matter, studies of this issue have found

that people become very uncomfortable with a rise of a single degree in their core temperature. Because significant increases in core heat can result in unconsciousness, the general precautions regarding body immersion in whirlpools also apply to pregnant women. Limit total time, and get out if dizziness or discomfort occurs.

2
PART

The Labor and Delivery Suite

5

Initial Patient Evaluation

TRIAGE

The labor and delivery area is not used solely to take care of laboring patients at term. It also serves as a sort of emergency room for pregnant women who are not in labor. With its fetal heart rate monitors and heavy staffing of nurses, this ward is well suited for rapid evaluation of pregnant women and for intervention, if necessary. **PEARL: When a patient presents to labor and delivery, her disposition depends on two things: (1) estimated gestational age (EGA) and (2) presenting complaint.**

Gestational Age

If the estimated gestational age is equal to or greater than 36 weeks, an intern or junior resident can evaluate the patient. If it is less than 36 weeks, however, consultation should be obtained.

Presenting Complaint in Term Patient

Patients at term usually come to labor and delivery for one of two reasons: **contractions** or **ruptured membranes.** Obviously, those with a question of ruptured membranes who are not contracting do not need to be seen as quickly as those with strong contractions.

ADMITTING WORK-UP

Requirements for this document vary among institutions. The history and physical outlined below are examples of what information is considered relevant in the work-up. In principle, a complete medical history is obtained at the first prenatal visit, so this history should not contain many surprises. It is acceptable to obtain most of the history from the prenatal record, although the important points should be double-checked with the patient.

For women in advanced labor who are in much pain, some of the information may be skipped. As an example, if someone is barely able to talk and already 5 cm dilated, it does not seem worthwhile to zealously pursue the accuracy of due date by obtaining a rigorous menstrual history. Also, many hospitals have abbreviated forms that make the admission work-up easier. The example below is rather detailed, and both time and the patient's discomfort may not permit a perfect document on every occasion.

History

Chief Complaint

Contractions and/or spontaneous rupture of membranes (SROM).

History of Present Illness

Ms. _____ is a (age), (race), G _____ P _____ (Term-Preterm-Abortion-Living), LMP _____, EDC _____ [by dates, exam, ultrasound (include those that are appropriate)] who presents to labor and delivery at _____ weeks complaining of _____. [The second sentence summarizes the membrane status and contraction pattern (always indicate the time of ruptured membranes).] She has gained _____ pounds during an uncomplicated pregnancy (**or** a pregnancy complicated by _____).

Prenatal Labs

Rubella titer (>1.0 or $>1:8$ shows immunity)
Blood type and Rh
Antibody screen
Other relevant positives or negatives
Ultrasound findings (if obtained)

Past Medical History

Hospitalizations, surgery, accidents
Medications
Allergies
Menstrual history: It is important to document whether regular or not when there is a question about the gestational age. Last oral contraceptive use, if relevant. Pill use within 3 to 6 months of the last menstrual period can delay ovulation and throw off dates.

Past Obstetrical History

Include maternal age plus gestational age, sex, weight, and route of delivery for each birth, along with complications. This can often be copied from the prenatal record without troubling the laboring mother.

Social History

Smoking, alcohol, illicit drug use, who is in the household, and occupation.

Family History

Be brief; defer if pressed for time. Include only relevant details (diabetes, hypertension, history of twinning, etc.). Again, this can usually be obtained from the prenatal record.

Review of Systems

Only relevant positive anwers.

Exam (Example)

Vitals

Pupils: equal and reactive to light accommodation
Throat: without erythema
Neck: without adenopathy, thyromegaly
Lungs: clear
Heart: RRR; S_1, S_2 with I/VI systolic murmur along the left sternal border
Back: without costovertebral angle tenderness
Abdomen:

  Fundal height (FH) = _____ cm.
  Estimated fetal weight (EFW) = _____.
  Fetal heart tones (FHTs) = _____.
  Contractions every _____ minutes (by palpation or monitor—indicate which).
  Draw a picture of the fetus, indicating head and back location. Be circumspect before drawing anything other than vertex. Put an *X* in the location of the fetal heart tones. Be sure to note the presence of any abdominal scars.

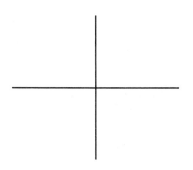

Pelvic:

Dilatation: Between closed and 10 cm (also known as complete).

Effacement: The normal cervix is 2 to 3 cm long. Thickness is expressed as %. A completely thinned out cervix is 100% effaced.

Station: Distance in centimeters between the lowest bony portion of the fetus and the maternal ischial spines. Generally, the distance is expressed as a number between −5 (above the spines) and +5 (below the spines). For clarity, the station is often given as numerator divided by 5, to distinguish this from the former nomenclature in which the station was described in thirds.

Presenting part: If anything other than vertex is suspected, consultation should be obtained.

Note: When the cervix is dilated enough, usually by 5 cm, it should be possible to feel the sutures and thus also indicate position (orientation of the presenting part).

Status of membranes: Either intact or ruptured. There are three common methods of determining that membranes are ruptured:

1. Fluid gushing from vagina (indicate whether clear or meconium-stained)
2. Nitrazine positive (amniotic fluid has a pH between 7.1 and 7.4, whereas 90% of women

will have acidic urine, thus allowing nitrazine paper to help distinguish between them)
3. Presence of ferning. Occasionally, cervical mucus can fern (adopt a crystal-like structure resembling the branches of a Christmas tree), so it is important to collect fluid from the posterior vault rather than the cervix itself.

Lower extremities:

Deep tendon reflexes (DTRs): (Note: Patients in labor normally have slightly increased DTRs, and up to two beats of clonus is considered normal. Up to 75% of pregnant women develop ankle edema at some point.)

Clonus

Edema

Calf tenderness

Impression

Patient is a ___ -year-old, (race), G ___ P ___ female at ___ weeks who presents to labor and delivery. . . .

Plan

Admit. Monitor. Anticipate spontaneous vaginal birth. . . . It is helpful to check with the decision maker (attending or experienced resident) before committing a plan to paper if there is question about the proper course of action.

TIPS ON DOING THE WORK-UP

PEARL: The key to being proficient in labor and delivery is to focus on brevity, completeness, and speed in performing admitting histories and physicals. Ideally, nothing should be written that is not immediately relevant, but nothing important should be left out. This is a skill that can only be obtained through experience.

Most of the history can be obtained from the nurse's admitting notes and the prenatal record. Obtaining the information this way is faster and spares the patient repetitive questioning at a time when she is in pain. It is also faster to record the history directly on paper as it is being obtained. Leave a few blank lines for filling in all the specifics of the history of present illness that can be done after you see the patient. On the physical exam, the two most important aspects that require completeness are the abdominal and pelvic exams.

CONTROVERSY: Some parts of the usual history and physical are unnecessary in examining a patient in labor. Specifically, the breast exam on a patient in labor is often unreliable. Laboriously recording all of the prenatal labs such as the serology and Pap smear also seems to be a fruitless waste of time. All of these items are addressed in advance of labor or in the postpartum period and are rarely relevant to the management of labor.

In this sample history and physical, I have omitted items that I consider unnecessary. Admittedly, my opinions about what is important and unimportant in the work-up are not universally shared. In the absence of an explicit policy, the guidelines offered here are a good starting point.

NOTIFYING THE APPROPRIATE PHYSICIAN OF THE PATIENT'S VISIT TO LABOR AND DELIVERY

This procedure varies by institution. In most cases, private obstetricians like to be called (day or night) with the initial evaluation of their patients. They also usually like to be notified before any pain medication is administered to their patients. They need to be kept up to date on the progress of labor so that they can have time to get to the hospital for the delivery. Again, policies about consultation with private physicians vary among hospitals and individual attending physicians. Consultation with more experienced physicians is not irresponsible or a sign of poor judgment. Lack of authorization for specific actions, however, is to be avoided. Nurses can be a good source of practical advice. When in doubt, call.

6

Care of the Laboring Patient

NORMAL AND ABNORMAL PROGRESS IN LABOR

In predicting the length of labor, it is important to keep in mind some basic definitions and concepts. First, obstetrical labor is not merely the occurrence of contractions but rather the progressive effacement and dilatation of the cervix in the presence of regular contractions. Contractions without at least some initial dilatation are not labor. The diagnosis of labor is necessarily a retrospective one because it is not always easy to distinguish between those having contractions and those having contractions that will lead to dilatation.

Most of the information about the length of normal labors and, indeed, the so-called labor curve itself comes from investigations conducted by Emanuel Friedman. Thus, the frequent references to the *Friedman curve* in the labor suite. A more thorough discussion of labor can be found in Friedman's book, *Labor: Clinical Evaluation and Management.*

Important Definitions

FIRST STAGE. This stage begins with cervical effacement and dilatation and ends with complete dilatation.

The first stage is further divided into a **latent phase** and an **active phase.** The latent phase begins with cervical change in the presence of regular contractions. The active phase that follows begins with an increasing rate of cervical dilatation. As with labor itself, these divisions of the first stage are retrospective diagnoses. In most women, the latent phase ends and the active phase begins at 4 cm dilatation.

SECOND STAGE. This stage begins with complete dilatation and ends with the birth of the baby. Mothers push during this stage.

THIRD STAGE. This stage ends with the delivery of the placenta.

Orientation of Fetus with Descent

At term, 96% to 97% of fetuses present head first. Of those in cephalic presentation, 95% emerge as occiput anterior. That is, the back of the fetal head is rotated anteriorly with respect to the maternal pelvis. Occiput anterior fetuses emerge with their face toward the mother's rectum. Occiput posterior babies are born facing the symphysis pubis and are also known as *sunny-side up* babies. Labor, particularly the second stage, often can take longer with such *posterior* babies. There is a widespread belief that *back labor,* in which the center of pain is located in the lower back, is more frequent with occiput posterior fetuses, although the evidence for this belief is largely anecdotal.

As labor progresses, a change in the orientation of the sutures can often be noted. With descent, the fetus will change from transverse (facing one maternal hip or the other) to anterior (facing the buttocks).

Limits of Normal

The following limits are prescribed by Friedman. It is critical to realize that these numbers are **not** averages but limits of normal. **PEARL: A given portion of labor is accomplished by 95% of laboring women within the time interval in the following list.**

First Labors

First stage:

Latent phase 20.1 hours (mean 6.4 hours)
Active phase 11.7 hours (mean 4.6 hours)
  Maximum dilatation >1.2 cm/hr (mean 3 cm/hr)
  Maximum descent >1 cm/hr (mean 3.3 cm/hr)

Second stage:

2.9 hours

Second Labors

First stage:

Latent phase 13.6 hours (mean 4.8 hours)
Active phase 5.2 hours (mean 2.4 hours)
  Maximum dilatation >1.5 cm/hr (mean 5.7 cm/hr)
  Maximum descent >2.1 cm/hr (mean 6.6 cm/hr)

Second stage:
1.1 hour

These normative times were in women who did not receive epidural anesthesia.

CONTROVERSY: It is generally thought that epidural anesthesia can lengthen labor, but the data are limited and contradictory.

Of course, dilatation is not the only parameter to measure in labor. Complete effacement is usually accomplished by 4 to 5 cm of dilatation. More important, the presenting part must descend at some point, or the baby will not be born. Women in their first labors will often have the presenting part engaged (at zero station) early in labor or before the onset of regular contractions. Women with subsequent labors will begin with the presenting part still high in the pelvis. In these women, it is not unusual for the head to be relatively high with complete dilatation.

Treatment of Abnormal Labor Patterns

Prolonged Latent Phase

Oxytocin infusion and narcotic sedation are both effective in ending an abnormally long latent phase, although oxytocin is somewhat faster. Amniotomy (artificial rupture of membranes) does not seem to be of benefit, although many believe that it is, in spite of the data. A prolonged latent phase has not been associated with an increased incidence of subsequent labor abnormalities or a detrimental perinatal outcome.

Protracted Active Phase

The contractions may not be effective enough. Alternatively, the baby can be relatively large or poorly positioned. In general, the approach to the evaluation and treatment of a protracted active phase of labor is similar to that of arrested labor, as described in the next section.

Arrested Active Phase

PEARL: There are basically only two reasons for a complete halt of progress in labor: poor contractions or cephalopelvic disproportion.

At this point, it is worth discussing *the three Ps.* This concept seems to be universally taught to all medical students and has remained unchanged for at least 100 years. *The three Ps* refer to the powers, the passenger, and the pelvis. Unfortunately, this concept does not seem to have any empirical grounding and appears to be the cause of much confusion. After delivering 2000 babies, I make no claim to be able to distinguish between a big fetus versus a small maternal pelvis. The idea that somehow we can distinguish between the two has led to some very peculiar outcomes, including cesarean sections before the onset of labor because the fetus is considered to be too big or the pelvis is considered to be too small. Perhaps the three Ps should be replaced with *the two Ps*—the powers and the progress.

CONTROVERSY: In practice, clinical judgments about the size of the fetus or the pelvis cannot be made reliably without observing the progress in a labor with adequate contractions.

The frequency of contractions can be assessed by an external tocodynamometer, but the adequacy of contractions can be assessed only by palpation, the progress of labor, or with an intrauterine pressure catheter (IUPC, described later). The minimal strength of an effective contraction is thought to be in the range of 40 mm Hg. The normal resting tone for the uterus is under 20 mm Hg.

In most labors, contractions occur every 2 to 4 minutes. Oxytocin can be used if the contractions are not frequent or strong enough. On the other hand, contractions that are too frequent may compromise uteroplacental blood flow. This *tachysys-*

tole, or five or more contractions in 10 minutes, can be treated with hydration, lateral decubitus positioning of the patient, and oxygen. Tachysystole, however, does not always need treatment and can occasionally be observed in naturally occurring labors resulting in healthy newborns.

CONTROVERSY: In the face of fetal compromise, some obstetricians use tocolytics such as magnesium or terbutaline to space out such contractions, but there is a lack of data demonstrating that this treatment is effective. The little evidence that supports this practice has generally focused on the treatment of nonreassuring fetal heart rate tracings rather than the treatment of tachysystole per se.

In assessing the sufficiency of contractions during labor, it has been generally recognized that contractions must reach at least 40 mm Hg to result in steady progress. An alternative method of assessment is to quantify uterine contractions in Montevideo units. This is determined by adding the sums of the peak pressure change achieved by each contraction in 10 minutes. **PEARL: A minimal level of 200 Montevideo units has been adopted by the American College of Obstetricians and Gynecologists as being the necessary contraction strength and frequency before considering a cesarean section for cephalopelvic disproportion (CPD).** It should be noted, though, that the contraction strength and frequency during labors resulting in vaginal births has been found to be so variable that it has been difficult to provide quantitative limits of successful labors.

CONTROVERSY: If the contractions have proved to be adequate by an IUPC and no descent or dilatation has been made over 2 hours, the diagnosis of CPD can be made. Some recent studies have suggested that the rate of vaginal births can be increased if the period of arrest in the face of adequate contractions is allowed to persist beyond 2 hours, but no consensus exists as yet.

The treatment for CPD is cesarean section. There are several important caveats to bear in mind. First, CPD before 4 cm dilatation is achieved is unusual, and it is important to be sure that lack of expected progress is not merely due to the fact that the patient is in the latent phase of labor. Furthermore, the diagnosis of CPD is more reliably assigned if the presenting part is definitely "stuck." If descent or dilatation has occurred over 2 hours, the fetus may still be born vaginally.

The diagnosis of arrested active phase is not as easy to make in practice as it might sound. As the fetus descends, the head undergoes molding. In some cases, the head may actually be "stuck" but may undergo enough molding to give the false appearance of progress. Furthermore, caput (scalp edema) may develop and also give the illusion of progress. The presence of significant edema and molding on pelvic exam should increase the suspicion of possible CPD.

CONTROVERSY: CPD is a diagnosis made on the empirical observation of labor. It cannot be reliably predicted from x-ray or ultrasound measurements of either the maternal pelvis or the fetus. There may be some exceptions to this general rule, such as the safety of vaginal birth for fetuses over 4500 g in diabetic mothers. Yet the term CPD has no universally accepted definition. Many obstetricians substitute the term failure to progress, although this term also has no clear definition. Perhaps the best way to think of CPD is to view it as a reference to the fact that the fetal skeleton cannot pass through the maternal skeleton (in vertex presentation). This concept eliminates speculation about whether the fetus is too big or the pelvis is too small, or whether the fetus is malrotated.

If the fetus is occiput posterior or asynclitic (head tilted awkwardly in the sagittal plane), is the position the cause of the failed progress, or did the fetus end up in this position because it was the easiest fit in the first place? At the present time, the answer is unknowable. A fetus who is not born despite adequate contractions may be thought of as having CPD—its skeleton simply could not pass through the maternal skeleton.

Recent evidence has suggested that the prognosis for vaginal delivery in subsequent pregnancies differs according to whether arrest of labor occurs during the first or second stage. Those who make it to the second stage of labor but fail to deliver seem to have a worse prognosis in future pregnancies than those who experience an earlier lack of progress.

Transfer of Patient to Delivery Room

In response to consumer demand, many hospitals have designed their rooms to be both a labor room and a delivery room. For those with the more traditional division between the two functions, a question frequently asked is, "When should the patient be moved to the delivery room?" The objective is to have the laboring patient in the delivery room 10 to 15 minutes in advance of the birth so that the delivery equipment can be prepared and the obstetrician can scrub. For women undergoing their first labors, the transfer should take place when the fetus is crowning—that is, when the scalp is visible through the labia between contractions.

Women with subsequent labors are much more unpredictable and should often be moved to the delivery room shortly after complete dilatation.

Those with particularly fast labors might even be transferred when they are dilated 8 cm.

FETAL MONITORING

There are two techniques to monitor the fetal heart rate. External monitoring uses Doppler ultrasound to detect fetal heart wall motion. The internal method involves placing an electrode directly on the fetal presenting part to detect the QRS pulsing wave, as with a cardiogram (Fig. 6–1). This can only be done if the membranes are ruptured, so it is not appropriate for monitoring far in advance of labor.

PEARL: Three important features of every tracing must be assessed before the heart rate pattern can be

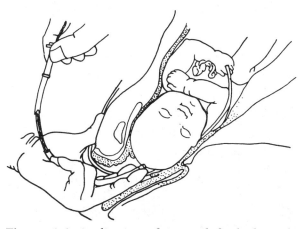

Figure 6–1. Application of internal fetal electrode (IFE). (From Freeman, RK and Garite, TJ: Fetal Heart Rate Monitoring. Williams & Wilkins, Baltimore, 1981, p 47, with permission.)

interpreted properly: baseline, variability, and periodic changes.

Baseline

This is the central *beats per minute* (BPM) value that the fetal heart rate oscillates around for 10 minutes or more. The normal range is 120 to 160. A baseline of more than 160 is a tachycardia; if it is less than 120, it is called bradycardia. Although a pulse of 120 has been traditionally considered the lower limit of normal, recent evidence suggests that rates as low as 100 are consistent with fetal well-being.

Tachycardia may suggest fetal compromise but not invariably so. The differential diagnosis of tachycardia includes prematurity, maternal fever, minimal fetal hypoxia, uterine tachysystole, drugs (atropine), arrhythmias, and hyperthyroidism.

Variability

Long-term variability (LTV) is an oscillation about the baseline that occurs with a frequency of 2 to 6 cycles per minute (Fig. 6–2). The normal amplitude is changes of 6 to 15 BPM (measured from peak to nadir of the oscillation).

Short-term variability (STV) consists of beat-to-beat changes in the pulse rate from one moment to the next. The normal amplitude is 2- to 3-BPM changes. This amplitude cannot be measured by most external Doppler devices because they add artifact (every plot pointed is an average of the last three beats) that appears to be STV. STV makes the heart rate tracing look "jiggly."

Decreases in LTV occur frequently and are most often due to sedation. Fetuses also have so-called sleep periods when LTV is reduced. These periods

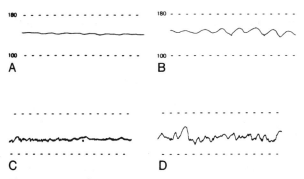

Figure 6–2. Short-term variability (STV) and long-term variability (LTV). **A,** Absent LTV, absent STV. **B,** Good LTV, absent STV. **C,** Good STV, absent LTV. **D,** Good LTV, good STV. (From Zanini, B, et al: Am J Obstet Gynecol: 136:44, 1980, with permission.)

can be quite variable in length. Other possibilities include early hypoxia, drugs, prematurity, tachycardia, tachysystole, anomalies, and arrhythmias. Decreases in STV are less frequent than decreases in LTV. Complete absence of STV is cause for concern.

Periodic Changes (Decelerations)

VARIABLE DECELERATIONS. Variable in shape, duration, and timing with respect to contractions (Figs. 6–3 and 6–4). The heart rate can often drop below 100 BPM and even 80 BPM. One classification scheme is given in Table 6–1. It is thought that variable decelerations are a reflex response to umbilical cord compression.

LATE DECELERATIONS. These decelerations are decreases in the heart rate that are late onset, mirror contractions in symmetry, and are repetitive (Fig. 6–5). They may often be very mild in terms of

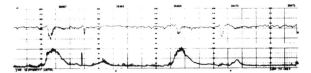

Figure 6–3. Tracing with mild variables. (Bottom portion represents contraction pattern.) (From Freeman, RK and Garite, TJ: Fetal Heart Rate Monitoring. Williams & Wilkins, Baltimore, 1981, p 71, with permission.)

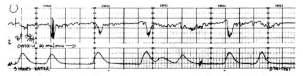

Figure 6–4. Tracing with moderate variables. (Bottom portion represents contraction pattern.) (From Freeman, RK and Garite, TJ: Fetal Heart Rate Monitoring. Williams & Wilkins, Baltimore, 1981, p 71, with permission.)

amplitude change. They also typically occur in the absence of accelerations. They are caused by uteroplacental insufficiency.

CONTROVERSY: Not all obstetricians agree about the definition of this term. The consensus appears to be that late decelerations assume significance only if they are repetitive, but there is debate about whether a single deceleration without repetition can be termed late.

As with baseline and variability, the interpretation of periodic changes requires experience and judgment. In general, the most troubling periodic changes are

- Repetitive, severe variables that are irremediable.
- Late decelerations that are irremediable.

Table 6–1. CLASSIFICATION OF VARIABLE DECELERATIONS

Beats per Minute	Duration (seconds)		
	<30	*30–60*	*>60*
>80	Mild	Mild	Moderate
70–80	Mild	Moderate	Moderate–severe
<70	Moderate	Moderate–severe	Severe

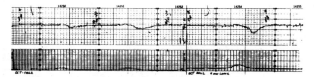

Figure 6–5. Late decelerations (also poor STV, poor LTV). (From Freeman, RK and Garite, TJ: Fetal Heart Rate Monitoring. Williams & Wilkins, Baltimore, 1981, p 68, with permission.)

- Prolonged, severe variables (lasting several minutes).

Intervention

Severe, Prolonged Variables

1. Change maternal position
2. Decrease uterine activity (turn oxytocin down)
3. Administer oxygen
4. Elevate presenting part
5. Prepare for cesarean section (patient should have an intravenous [IV] line)

One intervention that has acquired increasing popularity over recent years for the treatment of variable decelerations is the amnioinfusion, in which fluid is infused into the uterine cavity through an intrauterine catheter. The studies evaluating the benefit of this approach are decidedly mixed in their conclusions, and the apparent complications, including uterine infection, were not negligible.

Late Decelerations

1. Decrease uterine activity (turn off oxytocin)
2. Left lateral decubitus
3. Administer oxygen
4. Hydrate to expand blood volume
5. Prepare for cesarean section

Cesarean Section

The decision for immediate delivery on the basis of fetal monitoring is based on the periodic changes, together with changes in baseline heart rate or variability. Irremediable prolonged decelerations (for more than several minutes) or irremediable, recurrent severe variables or late decelerations that persist for more than 30 minutes are often indications for prompt delivery.

Scalp pH

This ancillary tool can be helpful in interpreting equivocal tracings. The membranes must be ruptured and the cervix dilated 3 cm before a pH can be obtained. Two samples are obtained per effort, if possible.

pH >7.25: Reassuring.
pH >7.20 but <7.25: *Preacidotic* (consider repeating in 30 minutes).
pH <7.20: Deliver promptly.

PEARL: Remember: Fetal monitoring more accurately predicts a healthy baby than a depressed baby.

The Limitations of Fetal Monitoring

New initiates to the world of fetal monitoring may be struck by the degree of disagreement among experienced nurses and doctors over specific monitor tracings. In fact, biomedical engineers have thus far failed to come up with reliable computer interpretations of fetal monitor tracings, in contrast to successful programs written to interpret adult electrocardiograms.

CONTROVERSY: Fetal monitoring moved from the laboratory into widespread clinical use before its benefits and disadvantages had been fully assessed. The methodology has simply not become as precise or predictive as was initially hoped.

During the initial research with fetal monitoring in the early 1960s, certain types of pulse patterns were associated with fetal hypoxemia in both animals and humans. At the time, it was thought that many cases of mental retardation and even perhaps cerebral palsy were related to events that occurred in labor. Because the initial observations seemed to support this idea, the monitoring technology spread from high-risk research settings into general usage, but it is now apparent that the initial premise upon which monitoring was founded was wrong. **PEARL: Of children born with mental retardation and cerebral palsy, 90% of cases are thought to occur before the onset of labor, as the result of injuries sustained by the fetus over a period of time.** Furthermore, among those few fetuses that are adversely affected during labor, a significant number experience sudden catastrophes that occur with little warning and leave little time for effective intervention.

In studies of fetal monitoring (started long after it was in widespread use), neonatal outcome has not been improved in low-risk populations. Furthermore, in comparison with populations in whom the nurse used brief periods of auscultation, the cesarean section rate increased. The initial premise was wrong, and in keeping with current knowledge, fetal monitoring in practice seems to be of no benefit to the general population. A small group of women with significant medical problems such as hypertension, heart disease, or diabetes may be an exception.

CONTROVERSY: With these limitations in mind, why monitor? Some obstetricians point out that it is cost-effective, because one nurse can remotely monitor several patients at the same time. Auscultation at 30-minute intervals for 1 minute during the first stage and at 15-minute intervals for the second stage has been suggested as an alternative by the American College of Obstetricians and Gynecologists, but this recommendation also suggests one-on-one nursing care. Perhaps once in a great while, the monitor tracing will suggest fetal intolerance to labor in a timely fashion.

MECONIUM

Meconium is a greenish substance consisting of desquamated cells and other materials that accumulate in the fetal colon. The passage of meconium sometimes indicates fetal jeopardy, although fetal monitoring and scalp pH determinations have supplanted the importance of meconium as an indication of fetal well-being. **PEARL: Meconium staining of amniotic fluid is common enough, occurring in perhaps 20% of labors, so that it may be considered a physiologic event.** Nonetheless, meconium in the airways can cause a potentially fatal pneumonia after birth. If it is thick enough, it may obstruct the airway and suffocate the newborn. As a result, the presence or absence of meconium must be noted whenever the membranes rupture (artificially or spontaneously). In most cases, the meconium is thin and does not prove to be a detriment to the neonate's health. Cesarean birth does not necessarily ensure protection against meconium aspiration.

In some medical centers, an additional person trained in newborn resuscitation is asked to be available in the delivery room, particularly if the meconium is thick. The obstetrician should remove as much of the meconium from the oropharynx as possible shortly after the emergence of the head (even before the shoulders are delivered). This should be done with both the bulb syringe and some type of stronger suction device.

CONTROVERSY: The traditional notion that meconium aspiration takes place with the first breath of life may be oversimplified.

PRESCRIBING PAIN RELIEF

Narcotic Pain Relief

The key principle in prescribing narcotics is "not too early and not too late." There is some evidence that narcotics administered during a normal latent phase may prolong labor. (Paradoxically, a therapeutic "sleep" with narcotics may truncate a protracted latent phase.) Of course, if narcotics are given too close to the time of birth, the newborn may have respiratory depression.

In practice, narcotics are not often given before the patient is dilated 4 cm unless sequential cervical change (indicating true labor) has been demonstrated. Keep in mind, though, that some women walk around for days or weeks dilated at 4 cm. As a rule, if birth is anticipated within 1 to 2 hours, only an IV dose is given (if anything). If birth is expected within the next 60 minutes, most physicians do not administer narcotics.

An example of a commonly prescribed dose of narcotic is hydromorphone (Dilaudid) 1 mg IV push and 1 mg intramuscular (IM). Table 6–2 compares various narcotic potencies with morphine. The IV dose provides relief in minutes but rapidly wears off. The IM dose provides longer relief, usually for 1 to 2 hours. Sometimes a higher dose given more frequently than every 2 hours will be required. It seems that each subsequent dose of narcotic provides less relief than the preceding dose.

Meperidine (Demerol) and Dilaudid both have peak action at 30 to 60 minutes after IM injection, although Dilaudid has a somewhat faster onset (15 to 30 minutes) and longer duration. Fentanyl is most useful as a fast-acting, short-lived IV agent.

Table 6–2. EQUIVALENT NARCOTIC DOSES (FOR IM INJECTION)

Morphine	10 mg
Hydromorphone (Dilaudid)	1.5 mg
Meperidine (Demerol)	100 mg
Butorphanol (Stadol)	2 mg
Fentanyl (Sublimaze)	0.1 mg
Alphaprodine (Nisontil)	45 mg

Butorphanol tartrate (Stadol) can be used either IV or IM in 1- to 2-mg doses every 4 hours. Two milligrams provides roughly the same amount of analgesia as 10 mg of morphine.

Occasionally an additional drug, hydroxyzine pamoate (Vistaril), is used with narcotics to provide additional pain relief. This drug potentiates the analgesic effects of narcotics and also has antiemetic, antipruritic, and antianxiety effects. Common doses range from 25 to 75 mg IM every 4 hours.

If a narcotic is given close to the time of delivery, the newborn may have respiratory depression. If the baby is not breathing adequately, naloxone hydrochloride (Narcan) can be given IM, and the baby can be assisted for a few minutes with a bag and mask. The usual dose of Narcan is 0.01 mg/kg. Because Neonatal Narcan is supplied in 0.02-mg/mL solutions for neonatal use, 1 to 2 mL IM usually suffices.

Narcotics commonly cause a decrease in the LTV on a monitor tracing. This fact is often used as a reason to withhold medication from women in whom there is some question about the heart rate tracing. It is important to keep in mind, however, that aside from causing respiratory depression following birth, narcotics are relatively safe.

The maternal side effects of each of the drugs are largely the same, although some patients will be adversely affected by one and not another. **PEARL: All narcotics can cause sedation and nausea.** Patients will frequently confuse a side effect such as emesis with a drug allergy.

Epidural Pain Relief

Epidural anesthesia is most useful for women in first-time labors. Epidural anesthesia tends to provide much better pain relief and is helpful at the time of delivery as well. As with narcotics, it is thought that administering an epidural before active labor can prolong the latent phase. Obstetricians vary greatly in ordering epidurals for those patients who request them.

CONTROVERSY: Some obstetricians insist on waiting until the patient achieves a certain absolute dilatation, such as 4 cm, but others permit epidural anesthesia to be given as soon as cervical change is established.

The technique of adminstering epidural anesthesia is highly variable among institutions and continues to evolve. The actual drugs administered also vary, although the most popular practice is to mix a local anesthetic with a narcotic. The drug can be administered in periodic doses, continuous doses via a computerized pump, or even a low, continuous dose with additional bolus dosing controlled by a patient-operated switch. A relatively recent innovation, which is more popular on the East Coast, is the so-called walking epidural, with which patients receive an initial dose of narcotic and anesthetic via a spinal, while at the same time an epidural catheter is placed for subsequent medication.

Although an epidural does not hinder interpretation of the monitor tracing, as can a narcotic, the epidural carries fetal risks. In particular, maternal hypotension with a concomitant decrease in uterine blood flow can occur. It is thought that this problem can sometimes happen even in the presence of a normal brachial artery blood pressure. The decrease in placental perfusion can manifest itself as significant, repetitive fetal heart rate decelerations. Fortunately, maternal hypotension can be corrected by either increasing IV fluids or by administering ephedrine 5 to 10 mg IV push. (Normally anesthesia personnel prefer to order this.) Caution must be used in administering an epidural if there is significant doubt about the heart rate tracing. A particularly common side effect is pruritis, which is generally attributed to the narcotic used. Diphenihydramine hydrocholoride (Benedryl) 25 to 50 mg IV or IM can be given for this side effect.

There is considerable debate about the effects of an epidural on the time course of labor. It appears, however, that epidurals tend to lengthen labor by slowing contractions—a situation often remedied through the use of oxytocin augmentation.

PROGRESS NOTES

Indications

It is helpful to write a progress note whenever the patient is examined, given pain medicine, or otherwise has significant intervention or change in status. Whenever the physician walks into the patient's room, he or she should initial the heart rate tracing for documentation of the evaluation. The policy on medical student signatures of monitor tracings varies among institutions.

Content

A standard note on a woman in labor consists of

1. Subjective: Her perception of contractions
2. Objective:

   Frequency of contractions (by palpation, tocodynamometer, or IUPC)
   Dilatation/ effacement/ presenting part/ station
   Statement about fetal heart rate and variability

3. Assessment: i.e., progress in labor, etc.
4. Plan: Pain medicine, continued observation, etc.

Chart Notations

In labor and delivery, there are several places to record exams. One is in the formal progress note section of the chart. Another is in the graph area where dilatation and station are plotted. Finally, the exam can be written directly on the tracing.

INDUCTION OF LABOR

Indications

There are a variety of reasons to induce labor. Three of the most common are discussed here.

1. **Elective.** Occasionally, the patient will have a strong preference for delivery before a certain date, such as job relocation of herself or her spouse. Elective induction also becomes a consideration for women at term with a history of fast labors who have advanced cervical dilatation with the current pregnancy. In these cases, if the induction promises to be a relatively easy one, it makes sense to induce labor rather than to risk a delivery en route. In any case, there certainly are situations in which a purely elective induction makes sense and poses minimal risks.

CONTROVERSY: One widespread practice that seems to make sense is the induction of women who are beyond their due date, out of concern that the fetus is growing larger and would therefore be more likely to experience CPD the longer one waits for spontaneous labor. There is at least some evidence that the opposite is true: Inducing patients for this reason actually doubles the risk of experiencing an arrest of progress during labor compared with simply waiting.

2. **Premature rupture of the membranes.** Roughly 10% of women at term will experience ruptured membranes before the onset of labor. Although 90% or so of these women will go into labor within the next 24 hours, the remainder will not. In some populations, particularly those women in lower socioeconomic groups, the risk of chorioamnionitis tends to increase over time. To prevent infection, many obstetricians will induce labor after some time interval (usually within 24 hours and often within 12 hours) if it does not begin spontaneously.

3. **Post-term.** In obstetrical parlance, this does not mean "past the due date," but rather at least 14 days past it. As the risk of perinatal morbidity and mortality begins to rise after 42 completed weeks, most obstetricians will deliver the fetus one way or the other between 7 and 21 days after the due date. Usually, this means the induction of labor.

Method

There are a number of different approaches available for initiating labor. The method chosen is highly dependent on an assessment of the cervix. **PEARL: The physical state of the cervix (referred to as *cervical ripeness*) has been associated with both the probability of successfully initiating labor and the length of that labor.** A semiquantitative method for assessing ripeness is the so-called Bishop score, which was first described by Bishop in 1964. This score assigns 0, 1, 2, or 3 points to five categories (Table 6–3).

In his article,* Dr. Bishop suggested that a score of 9 or more had a very favorable prognosis for in-

---

*Bishop, EH: Pelvic scoring for elective induction. Obstet Gynecol 24:266, 1964.

Table 6–3. BISHOP SCORE FOR ASSESSING CERVICAL RIPENESS

Category	Points
Dilatation	
<1 cm	0
1–2 cm	1
3–4 cm	2
5 or more cm	3
Effacement	
<40 %	0
40–50 %	1
60–70 %	2
80 % or more	3
Station	
less than –2	0
–2 to –1	1
Engaged	2
+1 or more	3
Consistency	
Firm	0
Medium	1
Soft	2
Position of Cervix	
Posterior	0
Midposition	1
Anterior	2

duction of labor. Currently, the chief relevance of this scoring system is to give the obstetrician some idea of the probability that labor will be easily induced.

For women who have a compelling need for delivery but an unripe cervix, there are two commonly used methods of ripening the cervix. The first is the insertion of laminaria (dried, sterilized kelp), which absorbs water and swells when placed within the cervix. The effect is to mechanically dilate the cervix 1 to 2 cm over 12 hours or so. A variety of synthetic substances for this purpose are now available as well.

The second method for initiating labor in a patient with an unripe cervix is the use of prostaglandin gel. Several preparations are commercially available, packaged as gels to be applied directly to the cervix or as a vaginal insert attached to a string for easy removal. The use of prostaglandins to ripen the cervix shares some common features regardless of the specific product. Generally, this method is used for those with a Bishop score of four or less. If the first application does not have much effect, it can be readministered, with the frequency and number of doses dependent on the specific product. Prostaglandins should not be given if the patient is already having frequent contractions that she can feel, and oxytocin should not be used simultaneously. These products often initiate labor as well as causing the cervix to ripen.

Most women at term will go into labor within 24 hours of artificially rupturing the membranes (amniotomy). This is also known as surgical induction of labor. The alternative is to medically induce labor with oxytocin, an eight-amino-acid peptide produced by the hypothalamus and transported to and released from the posterior pituitary gland. The chief danger of administering oxytocin is overstimulating the uterus. Fetal compromise or even uterine rupture may occur. However, with fetal monitoring and computerized infusion pumps, these hazards are rare.

There are a variety of protocols for using oxytocin to induce labor. Virtually all of them suggest increasing the dose of oxytocin every 15 to 30 minutes until the uterine contractions are 2 to 3 minutes apart. Some protocols start with an infusion of 0.5 milli-International Units (mIU) of oxytocin per minute; others start with 1 or even 2 mIU/min. There are also different ways of increasing the medication. Some hospitals double the dose at 15-minute intervals until 16 to 20 mIU/min has been achieved. Others increase it in either 1- or 2-mIU increments. In any event, it is unusual to require more than 20 mIU/min for a successful induction. Many protocols also call for either halving the dose of oxytocin or stopping it altogether in the event of significant fetal heart rate changes or tachysystole. Tachysystole may be defined as uterine contractions equal to or exceeding the resting period between contractions.

At the higher doses of infusion (perhaps 20 mIU and above), the antidiuretic properties of oxytocin become clinically relevant. If too much water is infused with the medication, water intoxication may occur, causing seizures and ultimately death. This is an unlikely complication, particularly with the limited amounts of oxytocin needed for most inductions.

CONTROVERSY: Is induced labor more painful than natural labor? Patients almost universally think so, although the medical literature is somewhat more divided. It seems that because the endpoint for the infusion, contractions every 2 to 3 minutes, may be somewhat more frequent than the average spontaneous labor, induced labor may indeed be more difficult. However, such labors are also probably shorter, and it may be that whether induced or spontaneous, the patient will experience the same total number of contractions. Although some data suggest that induced labor contractions have the same amplitude as spontaneous contractions, there may be a more rapid slope to maximum amplitude. It also seems fair to say that the latent phase of labor may be greatly shortened and that patients do not have a protracted prodromal period with which to gradually ease into labor. Also, in spontaneous labor, much uterine activity occurs outside of the hospital, before the patient is confined.

PREMATURE RUPTURE OF MEMBRANES AND INFECTION

With premature rupture of membranes (PROM), the risk of chorioamnionitis increases as time passes. The risk is generally small and remains small even with the passage of several days. Also, chorioamnionitis is largely cured with the birth of the fetus and rarely leads to serious complications.

Group B *Streptococcus,* however, can cause serious injury to the fetus. The incidence of this infection is 1 to 2 per 1000 births in the United States, but it may be further reduced through the more aggressive use of antibiotics. Group B strep infections can be classified as early-onset (within a week of birth) or late onset. Early-onset disease is characterized by bacteremia, pneumonia, and meningitis. The death rate can be as high as 15%. It is this illness that may be prevented in some cases with the use of antibiotics during labor. Late-onset disease is typically manifest as meningitis and is probably not affected by prophylactic antibiotics.

CONTROVERSY: The approach to preventing early-onset Group B streptoccal infections is still evolving. Two general strategies have been endorsed by the Centers for Disease Control and Prevention. The first is to perform screening cultures for all patients at 35 to 37 weeks and provide antibiotic prophylaxis during labor for those who test positive. The second approach is to administer prophylactic antibiotics during labor to those demonstrating clinical risk factors: ruptured membranes longer than 18 hours, labor before 37 weeks, maternal temperature of 100.4°F or greater, prior pregnancy affected by the disease, or history of positive vaginal or urine culture. Treatment prior to labor is not recommended because it is not effective in eliminating the bacteria.

The CDC recommends penicillin G, 5 million units loading and then 2.5 million units intravenously every 4 hours until delivery. Ampicillin (2 g followed by 1 g IV every 4 hours) is an acceptable alternative but its broader spectrum is thought to enhance the emergence of antibiotic-resistant organisms. For those allergic to penicillin, clindamycin or erythromycin has been suggested as an alternative.

7
CHAPTER

Procedures Performed on Laboring Patients

ARTIFICIAL RUPTURE OF MEMBRANES

Indications

There are two primary indications for artificial rupture of membranes (AROM): induction of labor and placement of internal monitoring devices. **PEARL: Of women at term, 80% to 90% go into labor within 24 hours after the membranes rupture (either spontaneously or artificially). AROM has not been shown to speed labor for women who are already contracting with reasonable frequency and strength (although it is often done for this reason).**

CONTROVERSY: Science notwithstanding, it is almost the universal belief of everyone who works with laboring women that rupturing membranes does indeed speed labor. In particular, women in second labors and beyond often seem to deliver very rapidly if their membranes rupture at advanced cervical dilatation.

Precautions

PEARL: The incidence of cord prolapse (an obstetrical emergency requiring urgent cesarean section) is roughly 3 in 1000 among women laboring with vertex fetuses at term. This is a small but real risk from AROM. As a rule, the membranes should not be artificially ruptured if the fetal vertex is not already well applied to the cervix to help prevent cord prolapse. This is a different issue than fetal station, because the fetal vertex can be at a relatively high station but still be in good approximation with the cervix. Of course, sometimes AROM is the only way to obtain critical information about fetal well-being. In these circumstances, the largely theoretical concerns over cord prolapse are set aside.

Methods

There are two ways to rupture membranes:

1. Amni-hook. Identify and stabilize the cervix with one hand, and snag the membranes with amni-hook in the other hand. Leave the examining hand in place for a few moments to detect any change in fetal presentation or station as the fluid leaks out.
2. The internal fetal electrode is very effective in rupturing membranes if the cervix is barely dilated or the membranes are tight over the fetal head. As the uterus contracts, the membranes will be sawed through by the wire and the drainage of the amniotic fluid will be satisfactory. It may take several contractions to assess adequately the amount and color of the fluid, however.

INTRAUTERINE PRESSURE CATHETER PLACEMENT

An intrauterine pressure catheter (IUPC) (Fig. 7–1) is useful when poor or abnormal progress of labor occurs. There are several commercially available catheters, all of which involve placing a microelectronic pressure sensor directly in the uterus. This technique simply requires zeroing the sensor just prior to sliding it into the uterus (the illustrated directions are right on the package). The catheter can only be placed after the amniotic membranes have been ruptured. It is often helpful to have the patient cough once after the catheter has been placed to be sure that it is functioning properly. The pressure readings, in torr or millimeters of mercury, are the same units used to measure blood

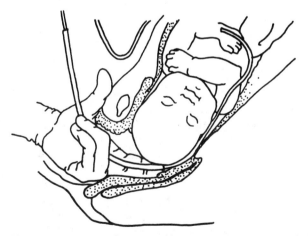

Figure 7–1. IUPC placement. (From Freeman, RK and Garite, TJ: Fetal Heart Rate Monitoring. Williams & Wilkins, Baltimore, 1981, p 45, with permission.)

pressure. Typically, the uterine resting pressure will be under 20 torr. With a cough, the pressure should jump at least 10 units. **PEARL: If the IUPC does not seem to be functioning properly, sometimes flushing with a few milliliters of sterile saline or water through the attached port is helpful.**

SCALP PH

Directions

1. Be sure that there are at least two scalp pH cartridges at room temperature and that the machine is on for 30 minutes prior to starting. The machine should indicate *standby*. Just before proceeding, slip a fresh cartridge into the machine, close the door, and wait until the machine reads *ready*. This takes about 2 to 3 minutes after inserting the cartridge. This procedure may vary among machines of different manufacturers and years.
2. There are two possible positions for the mother to be in: supine or lateral decubitus, with the buttocks flush with edge of the bed.
3. Open the kit, and put on sterile gloves.
4. Slide the white, plastic, truncated cone into the vagina.
5. Have the nurse affix the light source to the cone.
6. Slide the cone in far enough to visualize the fetal scalp. Press to form a seal between the cone and the fetal scalp so that amniotic fluid and cervical mucus do not enter the field.
7. With dry swabs, clean off the scalp.
8. Apply the silicone preparation with additional swabs. This helps the blood form droplets on the scalp rather than disperse.

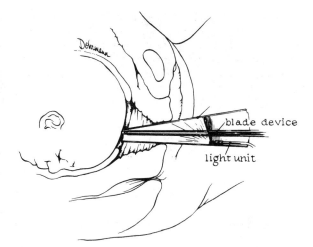

Figure 7–2. Fetal scalp exposed to hollow plastic cone; nick made in fetal scalp. (Adapted from Creasy, RK and Parer, JT: Prenatal care and diagnosis. In Rudolph, AM [ed]: Pediatrics, ed 16. Appleton-Century-Crofts, New York, 1977, with permission.)

9. Study the razor orientation on the long handle. Make an *X* in the fetal scalp with very firm pressure. This procedure may have to be repeated because the scalp is often soft and edematous.
10. With a long capillary tube, dab at the blood as it wells up (Fig. 7–2). While holding the tube transversely, dip the distal end of the tube into the clay and hand the tube off to an assistant. The assistant should slide the capillary tube into the upright receptacle within the cartridge. The machine will provide a printout of the pH within 15 seconds or so. A new cartridge should be immediately inserted to prepare for the second sample.
11. Repeat step 10. Observe the site to be sure that the bleeding stops. If necessary, apply pressure with one of the swabs.

8
CHAPTER

Vaginal Birth

TIPS FOR THE UNINITIATED

There are many texts on the so-called surgical management of a vaginal birth. Indeed, the public often looks at the unattended delivery as something of a medical emergency. **PEARL: In reality, very little assistance is required for most vaginal deliveries (Fig. 8–1).**

Novice Performing Delivery Without Immediate, Experienced Supervision

The instructions in this situation are quite easy. Do not break the bed or table, but do encourage the mother to push. When the baby falls out on the bed between her legs, suck the mucus out of the mouth and nares, dry the baby, and double clamp and cut the umbilical cord. Tears can be repaired after the delivery of the placenta, which usually occurs within the next 20 minutes.

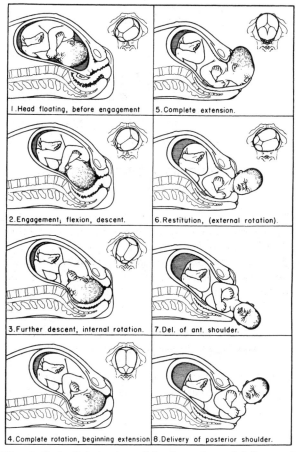

1. Head floating, before engagement

5. Complete extension.

2. Engagement; flexion, descent.

6. Restitution, (external rotation).

3. Further descent, internal rotation.

7. Del. of ant. shoulder.

4. Complete rotation, beginning extension

8. Delivery of posterior shoulder.

Figure 8–1. Orientation of the fetus through labor and birth. (From Pritchard, JA and MacDonald, PC: Williams Obstetrics, ed 16. Appleton-Century-Crofts, New York, 1980, p 397, with permission.)

Active Intervention

As the baby crowns, gently provide counter-pressure to prevent the head from popping out. If a tear seems likely, inject 10 mL of 1% lidocaine in the midline, taking care to protect the fetal head with the opposite hand. Even with the injection of just local anesthetic, it is advisable to aspirate intermittently to be sure that the drug is not being given intravascularly. During the next contraction, use scissors to cut the perineum down the middle (an episiotomy). If the scissors have one blade that is thicker with a rounder tip, use that blade within the vagina to minimize the risk of poking or cutting the baby. In some circumstances, the episiotomy should be cut off to the side (mediolateral) to provide the maximum room.

Occasionally, episiotomies (and tears) can bleed quite briskly from small arterioles. Simply put a hemostat on these discrete bleeding sites before or after the baby is born. **PEARL: No benefit to mother or fetus has ever been proven from an episiotomy, although it is reasonable to make this incision if a tear seems certain.** Repair of an episiotomy is often less uncomfortable than a more jagged laceration, which might need several injections of anesthetic.

As the perineum becomes increasingly distended, keep up steady counterpressure so that the head eases out. Also, use a towel or a sponge with one hand to support the perineum in the midline. It is helpful to pinch the perineum together to prevent tears or extension of the episiotomy.

When the head emerges, allow it to rotate spontaneously to face either thigh. Have the mother briefly stop her conscious pushing efforts at this point. Use the bulb syringe to clear the mucus out of the nares and oropharynx briefly. Before delivery of the shoulders, it is helpful to check whether the umbilical cord is around the fetal neck by sliding a single finger under the symphysis and palpating the neck. If the cord is there, it can often be lifted over the baby's head. Alternatively, it can be double clamped and cut on the spot.

After the mucus has been evacuated, the patient should resume active pushing. Gently guide the baby downward so that the anterior shoulder delivers under the symphysis (Fig. 8–2). The fetus should now be lifted upward so that the posterior shoulder does not lacerate the perineum. With the delivery of the shoulders, the baby will slide out quickly. It is helpful to grasp the newborn firmly but gently by the neck and both legs. If the baby is reasonably vigorous, he or she can be placed on the mother's abdomen, before or after cutting the umbilical cord.

CONTROVERSY: There is some controversy about where to hold the neonate in relation to the maternal abdomen and when to cut the umbilical cord. Some hold the baby below the perineum so that blood drains into the baby to prevent anemia. Others hold the baby above the perineum to reverse blood flow so that the newborn is not volume overloaded. It probably just does not matter for healthy babies. Also, the cord will stop pulsating on its own within a few minutes. Whether the cut is made immediately or with a delay is probably of little consequence.

It is important to dry the baby off in the first few minutes of life and to keep him or her swaddled to minimize hypothermia.

Some institutions routinely request that cord pHs be obtained to help define the status of the fetus at birth. Double clamp off a 6- to 9-inch segment of cord, cut it, and hand it off. Arterial and venous samples can then be obtained with a heparinized syringe. For mothers with blood type of O or for those who are Rh negative, an additional sample of

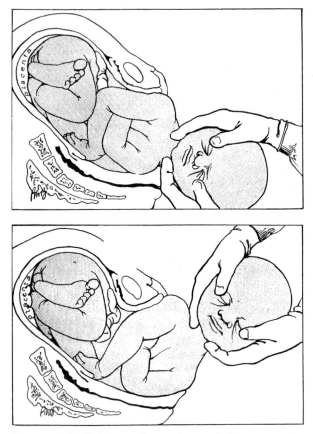

Figure 8–2. Delivery of anterior and then posterior shoulder (with *gentle* traction). (From Pritchard, JA and MacDonald, PC: Williams Obstetrics, ed 16, Appleton-Century-Crofts, New York, 1980, p 421, with permission.)

umbilical cord blood should be obtained to determine the baby's blood type, Rh, and bilirubin.

SPONTANEOUS DELIVERY OF PLACENTA

Spontaneous delivery usually occurs within 20 minutes, although it can take longer. If the placenta is not delivered within 20 minutes of birth, an experienced resident should be made aware of the situation. Once the placenta is delivered, it should be inspected on both sides for completeness and the number of vessels in the umbilical cord. As long as the placenta seems to be complete, exploration of the uterus is unnecessary (in most institutions).

EXAMINATION OF THE BIRTH CANAL

Following delivery of the placenta, the cervix, vagina, and perineum should be inspected for lacerations. With a sponge stick in one hand, insert the other hand into the vagina, applying downward pressure on the posterior wall. An assistant may also gently retract the anterior vaginal wall with an appropriate retractor. The cervix can either be grasped with ring forceps or blotted dry to aid inspection. If the cervix cannot be seen, it is acceptable to palpate it circumferentially to be sure that there are no major lacerations, provided that there is not excessive bleeding. Palpation is often faster and less uncomfortable for the patient.

After evaluation of the cervix, the vagina needs to be visually inspected, particularly in the area of the ischial spines, because tears are common here. The perineum should also be inspected, particularly in the area around the urethra. A rectal exam should be performed to be sure that there are no tears in the rectal-vaginal septum and to aid with inspection of the episiotomy or other perineal tears.

A first-degree tear is a break in the skin or mucosa. A second-degree tear consists of a laceration that extends into the deeper tissues. A third-degree tear involves the anal sphincter, and a fourth-degree tear extends through the sphincter into the rectal mucosa. Superficial tears do not need to be repaired unless there is bleeding that does not abate with pressure and time.

REPAIR OF A
MIDLINE EPISIOTOMY

An episiotomy is not as easy to sew up as one might first think. As the fetal head emerges, it compresses the posterior vaginal wall into the perineum so that they form a single plane. **PEARL: Following birth, the perineum and vaginal wall resume their initial spatial orientation so that the vagina again forms a 60° angle with the perineum.** The different planes and tissue layers can be confusing to those starting out.

The episiotomy can either be repaired with chromic (specially treated catgut) or Vicryl and Dexon (synthetic materials). All of these suture materials are absorbable. Chromic suture loses its tensile strength fastest—usually 50% by 1 week. On the other hand, it is usually gone by the time the woman resumes sexual intercourse.

CONTROVERSY: Some physicians suggest that there is more discomfort associated with sutures that dissolve faster.

Four layers need to be closed with an episiotomy. The steps below outline one approach among many.

1. **Vaginal mucosa.** A running suture of 3–0 gauge suture. This suture continues past the hymen out to the point where the tissue changes from pink to normal flesh tone. The suture is then not cut or tied but rather placed to the side so that it can be used subsequently (Fig. 8–3).

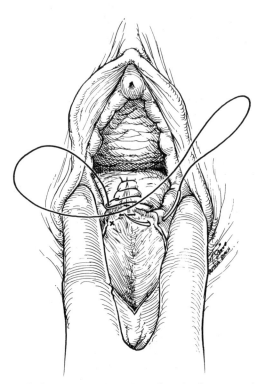

Figure 8–3. Reapproximation of vaginal mucosa (running suture). (From Pritchard, JA and MacDonald, PC: Williams Obstetrics, ed 16. Appleton-Century-Crofts, New York, 1980, p 432, with permission.)

2. **Deep perineum.** The shiny white sheath of the bulbocavernosus muscles is usually visible on either side of the midline episiotomy. Three or four interrupted sutures of 2–0 material are placed in this layer. Substantial bites of tissue are included on either side of the incision, because this reapproximation provides significant strength (Fig. 8–4).

3. **Subcutaneous perineal tissue.** The 3–0 su-

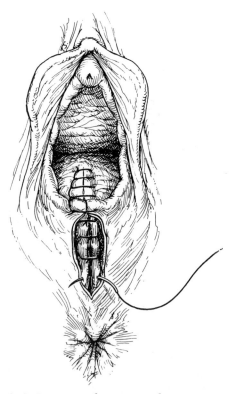

Figure 8–4. Interrupted sutures in deep perineum (bulbocavernosus muscle). (From Pritchard, JA and MacDonald, PC: Williams Obstetrics, ed 16. Appleton-Century-Crofts, New York, 1980, p 432, with permission.)

ture from the vaginal repair is brought out through the end of the repair underneath the skin. The running suture is then continued in the subcutaneous tissue in small vertical bites (Fig. 8–5). It is tied at the end of the perineal incision if a subcuticular suture is not used.

4. **Subcuticular suture.** This is a running mat-

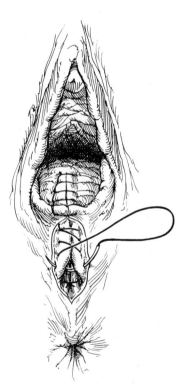

Figure 8–5. Reapproximation of superficial perineum. (This running suture can be a continuation of the suture from the vaginal mucosa repair. After this layer, the same suture strand can be used to finish the repair as a subcuticular suture.) (From Pritchard, JA and MacDonald, PC: Williams Obstetrics, ed 16. Appleton-Century-Crofts, New York, 1980, p 433, with permission.)

tress suture beneath the skin edge with 3–0 or 4–0 suture. Some obstetricians use this, and others do not. Those that do not argue that it is a waste of time, the perineum will heal just as well without it, and by placing absorbable suture just under the skin, the patient will experience more inflammation (and discomfort).

UTERINE ATONY

The most common cause of heavy bleeding after delivery of the placenta is uterine atony.

1. Massage the uterus firmly abdominally. If necessary, the massage can also be assisted with a vaginal hand.
2. Pitocin 20 to 40 mIU in 1000 mL can be run in at 200 mL/h (this may not be of immediate benefit).
3. Ergotrate 0.2 mg can be given IM. Elevated blood pressure is a relative contraindication to this drug.
4. Hemabate (carboprost tromethamine—a type of prostaglandin) can be given IM. It comes in vials of 250 μg. A common dose is 500 μg (two vials) IM. This dose can be repeated once.
5. Explore the uterus if heavy bleeding continues for more than 1 to 2 minutes and does not appear to be slowing. This procedure should be done by an experienced obstetrician, because it is easy to miss a portion of retained placenta.
6. If these maneuvers are unsuccessful, reinspect the cervix and vagina for lacerations.

OBSTETRICAL SHOCK

There are no principles unique to obstetrics here, although patients can deteriorate very quickly. Signs and symptoms of shock include pallor, clammy skin, rapid and faint pulse, and in advanced stages, decreased mentation or even unconsciousness. **PEARL: Blood pressure, pulse, and urine output are all critical parameters.** Blood should be drawn for complete blood count (CBC) with platelets and cross-match. Two large-bore IV lines should be established and a Foley catheter with a urometer placed. Junior residents should obtain immediate consultation. If a coagulopathy is a possibility, obtain a PT, PTT, fibrinogen, and D-dimer. **PEARL: MAST suits have occasionally proven helpful in cases of obstetrical disseminated intravascular coagulation (DIC).**

THE DELIVERY NOTE

The protocol for documentation of the delivery varies. Some hospitals even require that a note be dictated. In any event, relevant information includes the following:

1. Type of birth (normal spontaneous [without forceps] vaginal birth—NSVD).
2. Obstetrician (who was present).
3. Type of anesthesia.
4. Estimated blood loss.
5. Delivery of the placenta (spontaneous or manually removed). Be sure to record it if the uterus is explored.
6. Episiotomy or lacerations.
7. Mother's blood type and rubella immunity.
8. The baby: sex, weight, and Apgar scores. If the cord gases are readily available, these should be included, too.

The dictation that is mandatory in some hospitals restates the information presented earlier. If time permits, include a brief reference about the course of labor. Also indicate in the dictation a statement that the rectum was examined (and found to be intact).

POSTPARTUM ORDERS FOR VAGINAL BIRTH

Most hospitals have a preprinted order sheet. Below are some general principles.

1. **Fluids.** Mothers who do not have an IV in place are often given 10 U of oxytocin IM to help the uterus contract and reduce postpartum bleeding. For those who have an IV already established, 20 U of oxytocin may be added to 1 L of crystalloid and run at a 6-hour rate for one or two bottles. The type of crystalloid used ranges from D5 0.2 NS to D5 LR. After a vaginal birth, the IV line can be removed when the patient is stable and eating, usually within a few hours of birth. The benefit of postpartum oxytocin in the absence of excessive bleeding or uterine atony is controversial.
2. **Vital signs.** Every 4 hours for the first day. An example of guidelines for physician notification are for a temperature of 101°F or greater, a blood pressure of 160/100 or higher, and a pulse greater than 110. These suggestions are somewhat arbitrary and vary with each situation and patient.
3. **General diet.**
4. **Pain relief.** For vaginal births, Tylenol with codeine or Darvocet is often sufficient. An anesthetic spray (such as benzocaine [Americaine]) may be ordered to help with episiotomy pain, as well as sitz baths. Some doctors order ice water sitz baths rather than warm ones for the first 24 hours.
5. **Labs.** A hematocrit on the first postpartum day is usually adequate.

6. **Rubella.** Mothers not immune to rubella are traditionally vaccinated prior to leaving the hospital to be sure that they are immunized prior to subsequent conceptions.

7. **RhoGAM.** If the postpartum antibody screen is negative, RhoGAM is given to Rh-negative mothers with Rh-positive babies within the first 72 hours of delivery. Of patients who receive antepartum RhoGAM, 10% to 20% will have low antibody titers (i.e., ≤1:4) detectable postpartum. These mothers are still candidates for RhoGAM.

9
CHAPTER

Cesarean Section

HISTORY, INDICATIONS, AND TRENDS

In Caesar's day, a cesarean section was used to remove a dead fetus from a dead mother before burial. Prior to the late 19th century, the procedure had at least a 50% maternal mortality rate. Over the past century, the development of improved surgical techniques, suture materials, blood transfusions, and antibiotics have made this operation a reasonable alternative to vaginal birth in some circumstances. **PEARL: The ability to deliver abdominally has probably been a major force behind the 100-fold reduction in the maternal mortality rate in the United States over the past century.**

There are a variety of indications for cesarean birth. Common reasons include failure to progress, malpresentation (e.g., breech), fetal intolerance to labor, and maternal hemorrhage. Most of these indications are difficult to define precisely but generally fall into one of two categories: threat to fetal health or threat to maternal and fetal health. There are relatively few situations in obstetrics in which it is easy to say that a cesarean section is absolutely indicated. As an example, failure to progress may be appropriately treated with more observation, labor augmentation, or cesarean section, depending on the specific circumstances.

The cesarean birth rate in the United States has risen from roughly 5% in the early 1970s to approximately 25% by the early 1990s. There is much controversy in obstetrics about the appropriateness of this statistic. About one third of the increase comes from a higher rate of diagnosing dystocia or failure to progress. About 10% of the increase comes from the abdominal delivery of breech presentations, and perhaps 15% of the higher rate can be attributed to a growing propensity to diagnose fetal distress. Finally, approximately 25% of the increase in cesareans results from performing repeat cesareans, because there are more people who had the surgery in the first place.

One of the current controversies is the role of vaginal birth after cesarean (VBAC). The concern has always been about the integrity of the previous scar. If the scar breaks open catastrophically, a so-called rupture, the fetus can be lost and the mother can become quite ill. This is in contrast to the asymptomatic dehiscence, in which the scar separates without causing symptoms. Dehiscence can be detected on exploration of the uterus after delivery but this is no longer routinely done simply because someone has had a prior cesarean. The medical literature suggests that the risk of major maternal injury is the same or even less with vaginal delivery after a cesarean in comparison with the alternative of elective repeat cesarean. The risk unique to laboring with a cesarean scar is that the scar could rupture and compromise blood flow to the fetus as well as to the mother. This is not to say that obstetricians do not encourage patients to attempt labor after cesarean. However, those who decline do receive scheduled repeat cesareans.

CONTROVERSY: It is not clear that the increase in the cesarean section rate in recent decades is entirely without merit, although perhaps the magnitude of the rise might be questioned. The rate of difficult midforceps delivery has declined over the past two decades, and this may have played a role in increased cesareans over the same period. Perhaps some of the breech babies do benefit from surgical birth. In any event, the controversy over cesarean rates will no doubt continue for some time.

PREOP

Preparation

The following things need to be done to properly prepare a patient for cesarean section:

1. Nursing staff notified
2. Anesthesia notified
3. Written consent obtained
4. Magnesium citrate given (antacid)
5. Abdominal and pubic hair shaved
6. Foley inserted
7. CBC and type and screen sent off (sometimes Anesthesia will want to wait until the results are back). This step can significantly delay operation if not performed well in advance.

Important Preoperative Considerations

1. Know the **blood type** and **hemoglobin.** Be certain that the blood bank did, in fact, receive the type and screen (or sample for cross-

match). **PEARL: The only time you will need the blood is when the blood bank did not receive it.**

2. Know the location and reason for all abdominal **scars**—they will make a difference.

3. Know how much the patient **weighs** so that you know what to expect in terms of abdominal wall thickness. Pregnant women are difficult to judge in this respect.

4. Does the patient need prophylactic antibiotics? Certainly for indigent patients, **antibiotics** at the time of cord clamping should be considered for anyone who has been in labor with ruptured membranes. **PEARL: Before prescribing, be sure you know the patient's allergies.** The drug of choice is often an inexpensive cephalosporin such as cephazolin (Ancef) 2 g IVPB.

5. Does the patient have a history of **fibroids?** When in doubt, just ask the patient. A strategically placed fibroid can increase blood loss or make incision placement on the uterus more difficult.

6. It may be helpful to check the last ultrasound report (if available) for **placental location.**

7. Know if the amniotic fluid has been clear or is **meconium** stained.

8. Be sure to check whether the patient wants a **tubal ligation**—this is easy to forget. Patients on public aid need to have special government papers signed 30 days in advance.

9. **PEARL: If the cesarean section is for cephalopelvic disproportion and the head is tightly molded in the pelvis, consider asking an assistant to be available to help with the delivery by donning a sterile glove and pushing up from below if necessary.** This procedure requires preparation in advance. Often this problem can best be alleviated prior to the incision by gently pushing up on the presenting part to dislodge it slightly.

10. Obtain the **surgical consent.** (See Chapter 10.)

OPERATIVE TIPS

Entering the Abdomen: Vertical Incision

1. Stay in midline and stay in site of previous knife stroke.
2. Make long, even strokes with knife.
3. Fascia can be cut with knife throughout. Alternatively, a small incision with a knife can be made and extended upward and downward with Mayo scissors.
4. The two rectus muscles can be separated bluntly for a primary section. Often scar tissue will necessitate sharp dissection on subsequent sections.

Entering the Abdomen: Transverse Incisions

1. Start at 3 fingerbreadths above the symphysis to minimize the chance of bladder injury.
2. Scarpa's fascia often looks just like the rectus sheath.
3. Once true fascia is identified, you may put the knife down for a moment and bluntly dissect off fat and Scarpa's fascia. This dissection is neater and quicker on primary sections but not always possible on repeats.

CONTROVERSY: Some surgeons do not like this blunt dissection.

4. Enter the fascia by making two small incisions on either side of the midline, and gently connecting them with additional knife strokes using steady, even pressure.

5. Extend the fascial incision bilaterally with Mayo scissors.

   a. There are two layers. They can be taken down separately or together by undermining first with scissors.

   b. The lower layer may be closely adherent to muscle (which bleeds if cut). Also, the lower layer attaches to muscle more medially than the upper layer—frequently the incision on this lower layer of fascia has to be curved upward to avoid this muscle at the lateral aspect of the incision.

6A. **Mallard incision.** Cut the medial two-thirds of rectus muscles transversely. Do not cut underlying, closely adherent peritoneum. Frequently the muscles are tightly adherent in the midline, and it is difficult to separate them bluntly—make a mini-Pfannenstiel incision (by dissecting the muscle off the fascia).

OR

6B. **Pfannenstiel incision** (Fig. 9–1). After dissecting the muscle off the fascia above and below the incision, the muscles can be separated bluntly or sharply in the vertical plane (harder to do on repeat section).

Entering the Peritoneal Cavity

1. Make the incision as high as possible on the peritoneal surface.
2. The incision for a vertical or Pfannenstiel is vertical; for a Mallard, it is transverse.
3. Dissect in layers when cutting through the preperitoneal fat.

Entering the Uterus (Fig. 9–2)

1. Make the incision in the vesicouterine peritoneum reasonably far away from bladder (not too low).

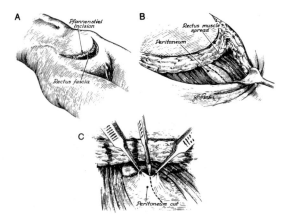

Figure 9–1. The Pfannenstiel incision. **A,** Skin incision three finger breadths above the symphysis. **B,** Rectus muscles exposed, separated in the midline and sharply dissected free from the overlying fascia, both above and below the incision. **C,** Incision into anterior peritoneum (entry into abdomen)—site chosen away from bladder at inferior aspect of surgical field. (From Wheeless, CR Jr: Atlas of Pelvic Surgery, ed 2. Lea & Febiger, Philadelphia, 1988, p 369, with permission.)

2. When dissecting the bladder off the uterus, remember that it is easy to poke a finger through the dome. Keep fingers well applied to the uterine surface, and move up and down—not side to side. If adhesions are dense behind the bladder, they may be sharply dissected with Metzenbaum scissors, keeping the tips pointed toward the uterus.
3. The uterine incision should be 6 cm long and made in steady, gentle strokes. A lap sponge can be held in the operator's nondominant hand to keep pressure along the incision. This method reduces blood loss over the incision and is more effective than aspiration in keeping the field dry. When only a few layers are left in the lower uterine segment, a single finger can be used to poke through. This poke should

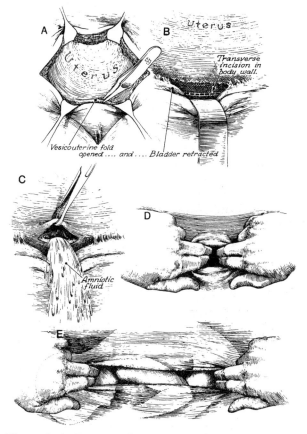

Figure 9–2. Entering the uterus—sharp and then blunt dissection. (From Wheeless, CR Jr: Atlas of Pelvic Surgery, ed 2. Lea & Febiger, Philadelphia, 1988, p 219, with permission.)

be straight through the wall—if it does not go through easily, more cutting needs to be done with the knife. The incision should not be bluntly dissected because this method often tends to dissect between the layers of the uterus and not through them, causing more bleeding.

4. The initial incision can be extended bluntly with fingers or with bandage scissors. With bandage scissors, care must be taken to protect the baby with the nondominant hand (babies have lost fingers when this method is carelessly applied). Also, the incision should be curved up as the lateral aspect of the uterus is approached to avoid cutting into the uterine artery. Many think that blunt dissection is faster, safer, and leads to less blood loss.

5. Occasionally, on entering the uterus, a sinus in the wall will be breached, resulting in heavy (and alarming) bleeding. In this case, do not panic or address that bleeding directly—proceed with the surgery. Because the blood usually obscures the field, the assistant will do what he or she can to keep the field clean. Because this usually is not perfect, you may have to proceed without ideal visualization. **PEARL: Remember to make the incision at least 6 cm long so that you do not dig yourself into a hole.** If you cannot see midway down into the uterus, continue gentle strokes and palpate the remaining tissue between every two strokes. Sinus bleeding cannot be effectively addressed until the full thickness of the uterine wall has been incised and the fetus delivered. At that point, a single clamp is usually sufficient.

Delivery

1. **PEARL: Be certain that your hand is actually in the uterus.** This point may sound obvious, but the

lower uterine segment is often thin and difficult to feel. More than one obstetrician has tried to deliver the baby with his or her hand outside of the uterus.

2. In delivering the baby, the hand should be under the head (sometimes a tight squeeze) before any upward traction is applied. The wrist should be kept straight, and the lower uterine segment must not be used as a fulcrum because this procedure will lacerate the uterus.

3. Fundal pressure is applied only after the head is within the incision.

4. Manual removal of the placenta during a cesarean section has been linked to an increased risk of postpartum endometritis. The placenta can usually be delivered by externally massaging the uterus. Nonetheless, it may still be prudent to explore the uterus, if only briefly, to be sure that the placenta has been completely removed.

Closing

1. There are six layers that can be closed: two uterine, parietal and visceral peritoneum, fascia, and skin.

CONTROVERSY: Some surgeons place sutures in a seventh layer, the subcutaneous (adipose) tissue, although recent evidence suggests that far from being helpful, doing this may increase the rate of wound infections. With a more critical, evidence-based approach to surgery, many obstetricians are eliminating closure of the peritoneum altogether and, in some cases, place only one suture line in the uterus.

2. For very heavy hemorrhage from a suspected laceration of the uterine artery:

   a. Use lap sponges to apply pressure to region of hemorrhage.

b. Obtain second suction and advise Anesthesia of greater than expected blood loss.
c. Very slowly remove packs from lateral to medial to look for bleeding source.
d. Ligate the uterine artery in two spots—low, near the top of the cervix (in proximity to the ureter), and high, where it anastomoses with the ovarian artery.

POSTPARTUM ORDERS

Vitals and Intake and Output

Vitals should be checked every 4 hours, and intake and output every 8 hours for the first few days. An example of physician notification orders are the same as those for vaginal birth: a temperature 101°F or greater, a blood pressure of 160/100 or higher, and a pulse greater than 110. Again, these suggestions are arbitrary and vary with each situation and patient. A physician should also be notified for output less than 250 mL in 8 hours.

Diet

Dietary recommendations vary among physicians. Studies of feeding postoperative patients suggest that the incidence of ileus and nausea are not greatly increased by rapidly advancing the diet. Still, some obstetricians will proceed slowly by giving only clear liquids on the first postoperative day and withholding a general diet until the patient is passing flatus.

Activity

By the first postoperative day, patients should be ambulated (although they are often quite reluctant to get out of bed). "Ambulate QID with assist" is a good order for the first day. Immediately postoperative, "Turn, cough, deep-breathe every 1 to 2 hours while awake" is also a good idea. For patients who received general anesthesia, the use of an "Incentive spirometer every hour while awake" to help prevent atelectasis may be a good idea.

Fluids

As a rule, 20 U of oxytocin are added to each of the first 2 L of crystalloid that are run at a 6-hour rate. The crystalloid chosen ranges from D5 0.2 NS to D5 LR. In practice, patients undergoing cesarean section are usually in good health, volume "overloaded" (from the pregnancy), and able to eat within 3 to 4 days postoperative. As a result, electrolyte balance, third-spacing, and precise volume replacement are not often of great concern.

Foley Catheter

A common practice is to remove the catheter on the first morning after surgery. Alternatively, the Foley can be removed a few hours after surgery. The logic for leaving it in overnight is to help the patient rest. Some obstetricians like to send off a urinalysis and/or culture and sensitivity prior to removing the Foley if the patient has not received prophylactic antibiotics. It may be wise to leave a Foley in place longer if the patient is receiving epidural or patient-controlled analgesia, because these methods of pain relief are associated with increased rates of voiding dysfunction.

Pain and Nausea Medication

Two methods of postoperative pain relief have largely supplanted the traditional IM injections of narcotics. The first, patient-controlled analgesia, entails the use of a computerized pump that the patient controls. Whenever she is uncomfortable, she can press a button and receive a small dose of narcotics IV. The pump has a lock-out mechanism set by the medical staff that prevents the patient from receiving too much medication.

The second method is that of administering narcotics through the epidural catheter. This can be done on a one-time basis before the catheter is pulled postoperatively, or it can be continued by computerized pump for several days.

Patient-controlled analgesia and epidural narcotics require less total medication than IM injections, so they tend to provide a better level of pain relief with much less sedation and nausea.

For those patients who require IM narcotic injections, hydroxymorphone (Dilaudid) 2 mg IM can be ordered. Heavier patients need more medication. These drugs and doses are examples of what can be used (also refer to the narcotic equivalency information provided in Table 6–2.) In the first 12 hours after cesarean section, the patient may not need much medicine if she has had epidural narcotics placed prior to the removal of the catheter.

Nausea can be controlled with prochlorperazine (Compazine) 10 mg IM every 6 hours, hydroxyzine (Vistaril) 75 mg IM every 3 hours (less often does not work well), or promethazine (Phenergan) 25 mg IM every 4 hours. Both Vistaril and Phenergan contribute to sedation and potentiate the effect of narcotics.

Antibiotics

Be sure to continue therapeutic antibiotics as indicated. Patients undergoing cesareans after experiencing fevers during labor are particularly at risk for developing postpartum endometritis.

Miscellaneous Medications

When the patient is taking in clear liquids, the oral medicines below are commonly ordered. Every obstetrician has his or her favorites.

1. **Tylenol #3** (acetaminophen with codeine), two tablets orally over 4 hours as needed for pain. Alternatively, Percocet (oxycodone with acetaminophen) or Percodan (oxycodone with aspirin), one tablet orally every 4 to 6 hours as needed.
2. **Simethicone (Mylicon),** 80-mg tablets orally four times a day as needed for "gas pains." Mylicon will reduce gastric indigestion but is of no benefit in abating pain due to small intestine peristalsis in the presence of colonic ileus.
3. **Triazolam (Halcion),** 0.25 mg (alternatively, secobarbital [Seconal] 100 mg or flurazepam [Dalmane] 15 mg) one tablet orally at bedtime as needed for sleep. May repeat once. Although these drugs may appear in the breast milk in small quantities, the infant is rarely affected.
4. **Milk of Magnesia,** 30 mL every morning as needed, or docusate sodium (Colace) 100-mg tablets orally twice daily for constipation.

Labs

Following a cesarean section, a CBC ordered on day 1 is usually sufficient. For patients with heavy bleeding, a pulse above 110 in the absence of fever, or a large drop in hemoglobin on the first check, it is prudent to obtain blood counts more often.

Rubella

Mothers not immune to rubella are traditionally vaccinated prior to leaving the hospital to be sure that they are immunized prior to subsequent conceptions.

RhoGAM

RhoGAM is given to Rh-negative mothers with Rh-positive babies within the first 72 hours of delivery unless already sensitized (with >1:4 titers).

THE DELIVERY NOTE

The note should include the following (time permitting):

1. Type of cesarean section—both the type of abdominal and type of uterine incision
2. Preoperative and postoperative diagnosis
3. Surgeon and assistants
4. Type of anesthesia
5. Estimated blood loss
6. Mother's blood type and rubella immunity
7. The baby: sex, weight, and Apgar scores. If the cord gases are readily available, these should be included, too
8. Any complications

EXAMPLE OF OPERATIVE DICTATION OF A CESAREAN SECTION

Name of patient (spell)
Your own name (spell)
Hospital number
Date of dictation and date of surgery

Attending surgeon

Assistants

Preoperative diagnosis

Postoperative diagnosis

Title of operation (be sure to indicate type of uterine incision)

Findings: At the time of surgery, the intra-abdominal contents, including uterus, tubes, and ovaries, were normal for a term gestation. A female infant with a weight of 7 pounds, 6 ounces, and Apgars of 7 and 9 was delivered from the left occiput transverse position.

Technique: The patient was prepped and draped in the usual fashion for a cesarean section. Under general anesthesia with endotracheal intubation, a vertical abdominal incision was made and the vesicouterine peritoneum was incised in a semicircular fashion over the lower uterine segment. The bladder was bluntly and sharply dissected off the uterus and retracted. A transverse incision in the midline of the lower uterine segment was made with a knife. The incision was extended upward and outward bilaterally with bandage scissors, taking care to protect the underlying structures with the opposite hand.

The infant as described above was then delivered. As the mouth and nares appeared, they were suctioned. When the rest of the baby was delivered, the cord was doubly clamped and cut, and she was handed to the pediatricians who were in attendance.

The placenta was then massaged out of the uterus, which was explored and closed with a single running suture of 0-chromic. The gutters, ovaries, and tubes were inspected and the pelvis irrigated with warm normal saline. The fascia was closed using simple interrupted sutures of 0-PDS. The subcutaneous tissue was dry, and the skin was closed using staples.

The wound was cleaned and dressed. The patient was then awakened and moved to the recovery room alert and in good condition. The estimated blood loss was 800 mL. The sponge and needle counts were correct at the end of the case. There were no intraoperative complications.

COMPLICATIONS

Although cesarean births may be commonplace, the surgery has real risks. **PEARL: As a rough guide, the maternal mortality rate from vaginal birth is 1 in 10,000; from cesarean section prior to labor, 1 in 5000; and from cesarean during labor, 1 in 2000.** Everything else being equal, a laboring mother is four to five times more likely to die during abdominal rather than vaginal birth.

These statistics can be misleading, however, because they do not take into account the indication for surgery. For example, a woman who has cephalopelvic disproportion during a prolonged labor has a higher risk of morbidity and mortality without the surgery than with it. Because death is still an uncommon event, it is more meaningful to review the morbidity rate from cesarean birth.

Blood Loss

The average blood loss resulting from a cesarean section is roughly twice that of vaginal birth—on the order of 800 to 1000 mL.

Infection

Infection is by far the most common morbidity following abdominal delivery. In some studies, up to 50% of mothers will develop a postpartum endometritis. This statistic is very dependent on the length of labor prior to cesarean and the socioeconomic background of the patient. A wide variety of antibiotics administered in the perioperative period for one dose have been shown to reduce the endometritis rate in patients at high risk (long labors, etc.). Perhaps 1% of those with endometritis will go on to develop septic pelvic vein thrombophlebitis, a more tenacious problem requiring at least a week of heparin.

Damage to Adjacent Organs

Injuries to the adjacent bowel and bladder are not unheard of and can require additional surgery to repair. Rarely, even the fetus can be injured during the uterine incision.

Pulmonary Embolus

Although pulmonary embolus is not a common occurrence, it is one of the most feared. Because patients with abdominal incisions ambulate less than those with vaginal births, an embolus is more of a threat. This is one reason that early ambulation is encouraged.

Anesthesia

Even among the doctors, there is a widespread perception that regional anesthesia is inherently safer than general anesthesia. This is not so. The mortality rate from both techniques is comparable and measurable in number of incidents per

100,000 (rare indeed). In the case of general anesthesia, the chief risk is from aspiration, whereas with the regional techniques, intravascular injection and subsequent convulsions and cardiac arrest are the chief problems.

10
CHAPTER

Informed Consent

Many private physicians prefer to obtain their own consent. For residents who must obtain the consent, examples for cesarean section and tubal ligation are given below. In my residency program, it was a matter of policy to write in the chart that the patient knew that a tubal ligation could fail. As a resident, I wrote the discussion down in the chart verbatim, although most of my peers were content with the routine hospital form for surgical consent. This type of documentation cannot prevent lawsuits. It can, however, help discourage them by showing the physician to be thoughtful and thorough. For those suits that are filed, a consent form can help your defense.

CONSENT FOR CESAREAN SECTION

The risks, alternatives, and benefits of cesarean section for _____ (give indication) have been explained to patient (and husband/baby's father). She (they) understands that the risks of cesarean section include but are not limited to

1. Blood loss requiring transfusion.
2. Infection prolonging hospital stay and possibly leading to other complications.
3. Damage to organs requiring additional surgery (either at time of cesarean section or in second operation) to repair.
4. Development of potentially dangerous blood clots.

All of her (their) questions were answered, and she wishes to proceed.

CONSENT FOR TUBAL LIGATION

The risks, alternatives, and benefits of tubal ligation have been explained to the patient. She understands the following:

1. The surgery is permanent.
2. Once in a great while, the tubal ligation may fail and a pregnancy may result.
3. Pregnancy following tubal ligation has a high risk for being a life-threatening tubal pregnancy. She will see a doctor immediately should she suspect that she is pregnant following this procedure.
4. The risks of surgery include but are not limited to infection, damage to abdominal organs, and the need for a blood transfusion. (These complications are admittedly rare.)

All of her questions were answered, and she wishes to proceed.

11
CHAPTER

The Newborn

Although care of the neonate is no longer a major aspect of obstetrics, newborns will occasionally need assistance during the first few minutes of life. With this in mind, some basic information about caring for them is in order.

APGAR SCORE

Often misunderstood by parents, the Apgar score (Table 11–1) is a formalized system to assess the need of newborns for medical assistance in the first few minutes of life. It is most commonly obtained at 1 minute and 5 minutes of life. Apgar scores are notoriously unreliable for predicting the health of the baby after these first few minutes. **PEARL: Only a small minority of infants with 5-minute Apgar scores of 3 or less are neurologically abnormal at 1 year of age.**

To judge muscle tone, merely move an arm or a leg and observe the degree of flexion. For irritability, scratch the soles of the newborn's feet and observe the response. The pulse is most easily obtained either by listening to the heart directly or by palpating the site of the umbilical cord entering the abdominal wall.

Table 11–1. THE APGAR SCORE

	0	1	2
Respiratory effort	None	Weak, irregular	Good, crying
Pulse	None	<100	>100
Muscle tone	Flaccid	Some flexion	Well-flexed
Color	Pale, blue	Body pink Extremities blue	Entirely pink
Reflex irritability	No response	Grimace	Cry

NEWBORN RESUSCITATION

What about intervention? The newborn should be dried off after birth and kept warm. Because newborns have a relatively large ratio of surface area to mass, they tend to lose heat very quickly. Keeping the infant warm during resuscitation efforts is particularly important.

Apgar Score of 7 or Above

The newborn does not require any assistance.

Apgar Score of 4 to 6

1. Continue stimulation by rubbing the feet, chest, or spine.
2. Be sure newborn is dry and warm.
3. Provide assistance with ventilation using 100% oxygen by face mask and gently providing

breaths at the rate of 40 to 50 per minute. Because the newborn has a small tidal volume (6 to 7 mL/kg), the puffs do not need to be very large. To reduce the chance of pneumothorax, avoid using great force in assisting the baby with the bag and mask.

4. Continue observing the other components of the Apgar, particularly heart rate, color, movement, and breathing efforts. Most of the time, newborns will become more active within a few minutes of assistance.

Apgar Score of 0 to 3

The neonate requires major assistance. When presented with a flaccid infant with few signs of life, most medical personnel experience a certain degree of anxiety. **PEARL: At this point, remember your ABCs—airway, breathing, and circulation.** Even babies who are quite depressed at birth will usually perk up quickly with a few minutes of low-tech intervention.

1. **Airway.** It is a common tendency to suction the baby vigorously, particularly when it is not moving much. Although suctioning is not particularly harmful in itself, it interferes with providing breathing assistance. Except in the presence of considerable meconium, gentle suction of the nose and mouth for 10 to 15 seconds should be sufficient.

   More important than suctioning is the appropriate positioning of the neonate. The head should be gently hyperextended to relieve potential soft tissue obstruction of the trachea (Fig. 11–1). This can be accomplished by placing a small towel roll under the baby's shoulders. It is not necessary (or desirable) to tilt the newborn's head as far back as it will go.

2. **Breathing.** As already described, 100% oxygen

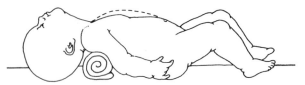

Figure 11–1. Position for keeping airway patent. (From Ostheimer, GW: Resuscitation of the newborn. In Ostheimer, GW [ed]: Manual of Obstetric Anesthesia. Churchill Livingstone, New York, 1984, p 337, with permission of the author.)

can be administered by bag and mask at the rate of 40 to 50 breaths per minute. Again, the key word here is gentle—puffs of 20 to 30 mL should be sufficient.

3. **Circulation.** If the pulse is under 10 for any length of time, cardiac compression should be initiated (Fig. 11–2). Chest compression for the neonate is very different than that for the adult. It is faster and requires much less force.

   a. Compression should be done at a rate of 120 beats per minute.
   b. The sternum should be depressed 1 to 1.5 cm.
   c. Use the second and third fingertips over the middle third of the sternum, or both thumbs while gently grasping the thorax with two hands.

Drugs and Other Resuscitation Techniques

There are two other things that can be done to assist the newborn: intubation and establishment of IV access for medication. By and large, the simple ABCs described earlier are sufficient for the first few minutes of life, and in most cases, they are all that is necessary. As intubation and IV access require some finesse and experience, they are beyond the scope of this book. Even so, a brief

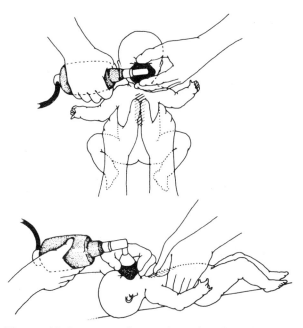

Figure 11–2. Neonatal CPR (two-thumb technique). (From Ostheimer, GW: Resuscitation of the newborn. In Ostheimer, GW [ed]: Manual of Obstetric Anesthesia. Churchill Livingstone, New York, 1984, p 336, with permission of the author.)

word is in order to give the junior house-officer an idea of the role of more advanced resuscitation.

1. **Intubation.** An endotracheal tube useful for the average term newborn is a Cole size 14 (with a tube diameter of 3.5 mm). A neonatal laryngoscope is required, and the head has to be moderately hyperextended, as already described.
2. **Circulatory access.** One of the most frequently used sites for obtaining access to the bloodstream is the umbilical artery. Although it is not an entirely benign procedure, catheterization permits rapid administration of drugs and easy access for obtaining blood gases to monitor

therapy. If the artery is too constricted at birth, the vein will occasionally be used on a temporary basis.

3. **Commonly used drugs and therapies:**

- **Sodium bicarbonate.** Useful for helping to reverse acidosis, the dose is 2 mEq/kg. It should be diluted with an equal volume of sterile water (with or without dextrose) and infused over 1 to 2 minutes.
- **Epinephrine.** Epinephrine is used to increase the heart rate and can be administered IV, or by the endotracheal tube. For the IV route, 0.1 mg/kg is suggested. The same dose can be given via the endotracheal tube but it may be diluted with 1–2 mL of normal saline for easier administration.
- **Volume expansion.** Dextrose in water (5% to 10%) or half normal saline at the rate of 100 mL per 24 hours. One bolus of 10 mL/kg may also be given. Alternatively, salt-poor albumin or even blood may be used (including blood collected promptly from the umbilical cord).
- **Naloxone (Narcan).** This is a particularly important drug for junior house-officers rotating through obstetrics. It can be administered IM and is contraindicated only in those with a known hypersensitivity to it (obviously not newborns). Mothers who receive narcotics too close to delivery will occasionally have depressed newborns. The dose is 0.01 mg/kg, so most newborns only require 0.03 to 0.04 mg. The reversal of narcosis is very rapid, with most newborns responding in 15 to 30 seconds of administration. **PEARL: It is important to keep in mind that naloxone has a relatively short half-life and can wear off before the narcotic has been metabolized.** Because respiratory depression can occur again, babies given naloxone have to be watched more closely in the first few hours of life.

3

PART

The Postpartum Floor

12
CHAPTER

Daily Postpartum Rounds

FOLLOW-UP OF WOMEN WITH VAGINAL BIRTHS

Recovery Period

Women are currently given 1 to 2 days following birth to recover in the hospital. Their exam should include reference to breasts, uterine firmness and size, and amount of lochia.

1. Breast erythema, localized tenderness, or nipple cracking should be noted.
2. After birth, the top of the uterus is commonly palpable at the level of the umbilicus.
3. Lochia (vaginal discharge) is generally bright red blood for the first few days and usually does not soak more than one to two pads per hour. Clots greater than 50 mL are abnormal. The most common cause of excessive postpartum bleeding is uterine atony.
4. **PEARL: Generally, the episiotomy does not need to be examined unless the patient has a fever or complains of severe pain in the region.** The epi-

siotomy may be seen by viewing it posteriorly, having the patient lie on her side and lift her superior leg.

Discharge Checklist

Prior to the discharge, the following items should be checked:

1. **Temperature.** If the temperature has been over 100.0°F in the last 24 hours, consider further observation. Examine the patient thoroughly for a source. The most likely possibilities are endometritis and mastitis.

2. **Rh.** If the patient is Rh negative, be sure to know whether or not she received RhoGAM. One injection protects against 15 mL of fetal red blood cells. If her baby was Rh negative, she does not need it. If the mother had a large fetal-maternal transfusion (unusual and will be noted in the chart), she may need more than one injection of RhoGAM. This can be determined by ordering a Kleihauer-Betke (hemoglobin acid elution) test, which can quantify the amount of fetal blood cells in the maternal bloodstream. Most obstetricians order this test only when a fetal-maternal transfusion is suspected, such as in the case of an abruption.

3. **CBC.** Patients who have a hemoglobin level above 7 are rarely transfused if they are not symptomatic. Oral iron is usually sufficient to reverse a postpartum anemia. Ferrous sulfate (325 mg) is often poorly tolerated. Depending on the degree of anemia, the nature and timing of follow-up, and the patient's preferences, smaller, branded iron tablets may result in better compliance. Also, the prenatal vitamins contain supplemental iron and should be continued in patients with blood-loss anemia.

For those with hemoglobin levels less than 9 g, twice-a-day iron supplementation is well advised for at least 4 weeks; those with hemoglobin levels over 9 g can manage with once-a-day supplementation. These recommendations are guidelines only and are somewhat arbitrary. Constipation may worsen with large doses of iron.

Instructions and Miscellaneous Considerations

1. **Sex.** Although some couples will not wait, it seems reasonable to advise abstinence for 4 weeks. This is an arbitrary period, but it usually allows the vaginal lacerations and episiotomy to heal enough to permit intercourse without great discomfort. Even so, most women will have at least some discomfort with the resumption of sexual activity. Also, some may notice inadequate vaginal lubrication. These patients should be reassured that this is a temporary condition that resolves within a few months. **PEARL: K-Y Jelly or other water-soluble lubricants may be suggested as an alternative.**
2. **Contraception.** Some centers will start some patients on oral contraception on postpartum day 14. The delay of 2 weeks is recommended to avoid the peak of hypercoagulability from pregnancy. An alternative is wait to prescribe the pill until the postpartum check-up. **PEARL: The estrogen-progestin pill may be prescribed to nursing mothers, but patients should be cautioned that milk production may be slightly decreased.** The progestin-only pill (Micronor, for instance) may also be given without an effect on milk production, although unpredictable bleeding can be a side effect.

   For those who are breast-feeding or do not want the pill, the condom is the method of choice for the first few postpartum months, because the diaphragm has uncertain effectiveness in this time span. An IUD can be placed during this time, although the manufacturer recommends that insertion not take place during the first postpartum month, to reduce the chance of uterine perforation.

3. **Driving.** Driving poses no inherent dangers to the new mother, but she may pose dangers to others in the first few weeks. Those with significant episiotomy pain may experience a slight hesitation in using the brake because of their discomfort. Mothers who are anemic or very fatigued may not be as attentive as they should be while driving. It seems prudent to proscribe driving for the first few weeks, although the advice should be individualized.

4. **Bathing.** Tub baths can be very soothing for episiotomy repairs, and mothers should be encouraged to use them. For those with cesarean section, many obstetricians prefer to avoid soaking the incision for 1 to 2 weeks after surgery, although there is no harm in getting it wet during a shower.

5. **Activity.** A good, common-sense rule is that "If it hurts, don't do it." The more patients move around in the first week or so, the more uncomfortable their episiotomy becomes, although activity will not slow its healing. For those who want to resume exercise, advice should be tailored to the patient's circumstances.

6. **Vaginal bleeding.** Vaginal bleeding can persist for 3 to 4 weeks, although it should not be heavier than a period. The passage of blood clots alone does not signify abnormally heavy bleeding. Women who have to change more than one or two pads an hour for several hours should call. It is reasonable to restrict tampon use for the first 2 to 4 weeks to allow the lacerations to heal and the cervix to constrict.

7. **Bowel care.** Most mothers are at least somewhat fearful of their first postpartum bowel movement because of constipation or the presence of stitches in close proximity to the anus. With the ever-shortening hospital stay, patients are frequently sent home prior to moving their bowels. Rarely, women can become impacted. To prevent this, mothers should be encouraged to take some sort of laxative such as Milk of Magnesia or bisacodyl (Dulcolax; two tablets) on a daily basis until their first bowel movement, and to call the doctor if they have not moved their bowels by postpartum day 5. Those who are having so much perineal pain that it interferes with bowel function might merit an exam to check for hematomas or infection.

Hemorrhoids are also a major source of concern, although they invariably improve at least somewhat with the birth. There are three steps for helping those with hemorrhoids:

   a. Add fiber and fluid to the diet to reduce constipation. Simply increasing vegetables is usually not enough, and specific diet additives such as Metamucil or Fiberall may be more helpful.
   b. Avoid traumatizing the area. This can be accomplished by minimizing wiping after defecation or by using soft medicated pads such as Tucks.
   c. Ease pain and swelling by using rectal suppositories after each bowel movement. A good over-the-counter drug is Preparation H. An alternative prescription medication is Anusol-HC, on awakening and at bedtime (and after each bowel movement). This product is a mixture of medications including a topical anesthetic and hydrocortisone.

8. **Pain medication.** Narcotic pain relief is rarely necessary after vaginal birth, although some

women with particularly uncomfortable episiotomies will benefit from it. Acetaminophen with codeine (Tylenol #3), two tablets every 4 hours, is often helpful. An alternative is 100 mg of propoxyphene with 650 mg of acetaminophen (Darvocet-N 100), one tablet every 4 hours as needed.

9. **Swelling.** Some women will notice increased swelling in their legs and hands during the first few days after birth. This is normal and is a result of fluid shifts following birth that resolve within a week by diuresis.

10. **Breast care.** See Chapter 13.

FOLLOW-UP OF CESAREAN SECTION PATIENTS

Progress Notes

The guidelines presented here are one approach to the documentation on a postoperative patient. The usual postpartum hospital stay following a cesarean section is 3 to 4 days. For the first 2 days or so following cesarean birth, progress notes should include reference to the following:

1. Vital signs and urine output
2. Breasts (lactation progress)
3. Lungs
4. Abdomen: bowel sounds/distention/tenderness/ uterine firmness
5. Incision
6. Quantity of lochia
7. Lower extremities: tenderness, palpable cords, edema

Following the first 2 days or so, the notes can be less extensive as long as the patient is doing well.

The abdominal exam and reference to the incision remain important.

Follow-up Labs

The labs usually obtained are a CBC on days 1 and 3 following surgery. Occasionally, a urinalysis and/or culture is obtained on removal of the Foley.

Special Problems Following Cesarean Section

Return of Bowel Function

The large intestine is usually the last to recover following surgery. Bowel sounds are generated by the small intestine as the postoperative ileus resolves. The first signal that the large intestines are working is the passage of gas. Bowel sounds are usually reasonably active by 24 hours following surgery. Passage of flatus is variable but usually occurs between days 2 and 4.

Obstetricians vary widely in their approaches toward feeding the postoperative patient. One common method allows the patient liquids with active bowel sounds and then a general diet following flatus. The IV is removed when the patient is tolerating liquids well, as long as she is not receiving antibiotics. Some obstetricians choose to feed their patients immediately with either clear liquids or a general diet.

Removal of the Foley

The Foley catheter is necessary only during the surgery to keep the bladder deflated. Also, many patients will have urinary retention during emergence from anesthesia. After this point, however, the longer the Foley is kept in, the greater the risk of infection. Generally, the Foley is retained for the first night after surgery to spare the patient the discomfort of getting up several times in the middle of the night to void. If the patient is not taking antibiotics, it is often helpful to get a urinalysis at the time of Foley removal, and then send a culture (from a refrigerated sample from the catheter) if the urinalysis suggests a urinary tract infection.

Staple Removal

This process, universally dreaded by patients having it done for the first time, actually involves minimal discomfort and takes about 60 seconds. Obstetricians vary on when they want the staples removed, but a common approach is to take them out on day 3 for transverse incisions and on day 4 for vertical incisions. Most physicians place Steri-strips on the wound edges following staple removal. The patient should be advised that the Steri-Strips are not holding her together and that those that have not fallen off in 7 days can be removed by tugging at both ends.

Activity

Thrombosis is a threat to an immobilized postpartum patient. Women recovering from cesarean section should be urged to begin walking on the first day postoperative (up QID with assist). They may also practice coughing and deep breathing. Those at higher risk for atelectasis (general anesthesia, vertical scar) should be asked to use an incentive spirometer every hour while awake.

Fever

Several causes of fever must be considered following cesarean birth.

1. **Atelectasis.** More common in smokers with a vertical incision and general anesthesia, it can also occur in nonsmokers with a transverse incision done under epidural. Physical findings are usually not prominent, although they may include increased pulse and respiratory rate and decreased breath sounds over the posterior lung bases. Atelectasis is usually not a cause of a temperature greater than 101°F for several days. Pneumonia must be considered should there be a high fever and prominent lung findings. In this case, a chest x-ray would be helpful.
2. **Urinary tract infections.** These are not usually thought to be a cause of fever unless the kidneys are involved.
3. **Mastitis.** See Chapter 13.
4. **Deep vein thrombosis.** A serious postoperative complication, deep vein thrombosis can cause fever but is very uncommon.
5. **Endometritis.** This is one of the most common causes of postoperative fever, particularly after day 2 or 3 postoperative. (See Chapter 14.)

13
CHAPTER

Lactation

Obstetrics is prone to fads, and breast-feeding is certainly not immune. A few decades ago, bottle-feeding was the rage, and now the pendulum is swinging the other way. Breast-feeding probably does offer some modest benefits over bottle-feeding, but formula-fed babies certainly can and do thrive just fine. **PEARL: Perhaps the most important consideration in counseling mothers on feeding their newborns is to avoid instilling gratuitous guilt.** Parenthood is filled with anxiety as it is, and pressuring mothers either to bottle-feed or breast-feed provides no benefit. For some working mothers or those quite anxious about it, breast-feeding will not enhance bonding.

BREAST-FEEDING

Breast-feeding has some health advantages when compared with formula use. First, it is probably superior to bottle-feeding in terms of transferring immunity and important proteins. Formula contamination and expense are also avoided. Because formula is somewhat higher in calories than breast milk, breast-fed babies may be less prone to excessive weight gain. Finally, for the mother who enjoys it, breast-feeding does enhance her relationship with the newborn.

As for breast-feeding itself, the sooner it is initiated after birth, the faster milk will come in. Frequent feedings, every 2 to 3 hours, are advantageous. In terms of technique, the baby should be held so that it does not have to strain for the nipple. Also, because neonates are obligate nose breathers, the breast tissue should not block the nares. To remove the baby from the breast, the mouth suction on the nipple can be gently broken by inserting a finger into the side of the baby's mouth.

It can take a few days for the baby to get used to breast-feeding, and mothers so inclined should be encouraged to persist. **PEARL: Babies normally lose up to 10% of their body weight postpartum, although they rapidly regain it.** Many drugs can be excreted in breast milk, but few of them pose a threat to the baby. Specifically, it is acceptable to breast-feed with most antibiotics.

LACTATION SUPPRESSION

The only widely accepted approach to lactation supression is the use of a tight bra and cold packs. Analgesics are frequently necessary because the resulting breast engorgement can be quite painful. The previous practice of giving high-dose estrogens in the immediate postpartum period did seem to make the process less painful but has been linked to increased risk of thromboembolism. Similarly, the use of bromocriptine (Parlodel) also promised some benefit, but it has been linked to an increased risk of seizures, stroke, and myocardial infarction.

BREAST ENGORGEMENT
AND MASTITIS

There is debate about whether severe breast engorgement can cause a low-grade fever. It is rarely a cause of spiking fevers of temperatures above 101°F. In contrast, if there is localized warmth, tenderness, and erythema in one breast, mastitis is a possibility, although this condition often occurs several weeks postpartum, after the patient has been discharged.

Patients with mastitis should be advised to continue breast-feeding and to use warm packs and acetaminophen to ease their discomfort. Although the milk itself can be cultured and gram stained, this is not always necessary in patients with characteristic findings. The bacteria often enter the breast through a cracked nipple. Common pathogens include *Staphylococcus aureus,* betahemolytic streptococci, *Escherichia coli,* and *Haemophilus influenzae.*

PEARL: The initial antibiotic of choice for mastitis is dicloxacillin 500 mg four times a day for 1 week. For those allergic to penicillin, 250 mg of erythromycin four times a day may be used.

Those who are not significantly better within 48 hours should be examined for a breast abscess. These lesions frequently require incision and drainage. Early administration of antibiotics is usually effective in preventing this complication.

14
CHAPTER

Postpartum Endometritis

RISK FACTORS

In some populations, as many as 50% of women undergoing cesarean section during labor have postoperative endometritis, although this number can be reduced to 20% or even lower with the appropriate use of prophylactic antibiotics. Endometritis following vaginal birth is much less frequent—on the order of 1%, and these infections tend to be less severe.

DIAGNOSIS

PEARL: Endometritis, the most common cause of sustained postoperative fever, is a diagnosis of exclusion. No reliable physical or laboratory findings are completely diagnostic. The uterus is always tender following cesarean section, and lochia can be foul smelling even without significant infection. The white blood cell count can be elevated up to 20,000 following cesarean section done during labor in the absence of endometritis.

The common practice is to exclude other causes of fever and then to initiate antibiotics. Often, with a temperature spike, obstetricians will draw blood cultures from two separate sites and obtain a urine culture prior to starting antibiotics, although these cultures rarely show bacteria. Lochia cultures are not usually of benefit. A CBC obtained within 24 hours of the first fever spike (before or after) is often sufficient. A differential adds expense and is rarely of diagnostic benefit.

When microbes are recovered, common isolates include the aerobes *Escherichia coli,* Group B betahemolytic streptococci, enterococci, and the anaerobes such as *Peptostreptococcus, Chlamydia,* and a variety of *Bacteroides* species.

TREATMENT

The most thoroughly tested and effective regimen for postpartum endometritis is a combination of clindamycin (900 mg every 8 hours) and gentamicin (1.5 mg/kg every 8 hours) intravenously. This treatment covers a wide variety of likely pathogens, such as gram-negative bacilli and anaerobes such as *Bacteroides.* In patients who do not respond, or for those who are severely ill, a penicillin might be considered for coverage against group D streptococci (enterococci).

As a two-drug therapy, gentamicin and clindamycin seem to be superior to ampicillin and gentamicin. Other regimens have not been tested as thoroughly. Alternative treatment includes single-agent therapy with a second-generation cephalosporin or with a third-generation penicillin (mezlocillin 3 g IVPB every 4 hours). Third-generation penicillins kill both group D streptococci and *Bacteroides fragilis.*

With gentamicin, some physicians obtain peak and trough levels around the third or fourth dose. If there is a question about impaired renal function, checking a BUN and creatinine before or shortly after starting treatment might be a good idea. **PEARL: An alternative dosing schedule of gentamicin that is less expensive and does not require peak and trough levels is 5 mg/kg once daily.**

For treatment failures, Primaxin seems to be a good first choice as an alternative to multiple drug therapy. Primaxin is a 1:1 mixture of imipenem and cilastatin, and it kills a broad range of pathogens, including *Bacteroides* and *Staphylococcus* species. The usual dose is 500 mg IV piggyback every 6 hours.

Pseudomembranous colitis can be a problem with any antibiotic. Diarrhea consisting of several loose stools per day warrants sending off a stool sample for *Clostridium difficile* toxin and culture, although the drug can be continued pending the results if the patient is not toxic. *C. difficile* can be treated with metronidazole 500 mg BID orally for 7 to 14 days.

One clinical sign carries weight over all others in determining the response to therapy—the maximum temperature (T-max) in a 24-hour period. As long as this value begins to drop within 48 hours of initiating therapy, the antibiotic regimen is not changed. If T-max is not improving after 48 hours of maximal antibiotic therapy, abscess or septic pelvic vein thrombosis becomes a concern. These conditions are both quite rare.

As a rule, the drugs are continued for a total of 4 to 5 days and for 24 to 48 hours after defervescence (depending on response and severity of infection). Although it is common practice in some institutions to discharge patients with a course of additional, oral antibiotics, the benefit of this treatment is controversial and should be individualized.

SEPTIC PELVIC VEIN THROMBOSIS AND PELVIC ABSCESS

If a patient's postoperative fever fails to respond to appropriate antibiotics, and a pelvic exam does not suggest an abscess, heparin is usually started. A bolus of 5000 or 10,000 U is given in 1 hour, followed by 1000 U per hour, with subsequent dose titration based on obtaining a PTT every 4 hours until it is one and a half to two times longer than the control. **PEARL: After the first day or so, the patient can be treated with a twice-daily subcutaneous dose of 1 mg/ kg of enoxaparin (Lovenox).**

CONTROVERSY: The traditional view is that heparin treatment in this situation serves both a diagnostic and therapeutic purpose. Recently, some questions have arisen as to whether heparin is actually more effective than simply continuing the antibiotics by themselves for a longer period of time. Nonetheless, if the patient responds, the heparin is continued for 7 to 10 days and then stopped without additional anticoagulation. Also, septic deep venous thrombosis should be distinguished from clots arising without prior infection in this circumstance, because most obstetricians would continue anticoagulation for several months with warfarin. Aside from controversy about the utility of heparin, the disease pathogenesis remains somewhat unclear: Is this a clot that became infected or an infection that led to a clot?

If the T-max does not begin to drop within 48 hours of beginning heparin, then an abscess must be considered. In this case, an abdominal CT or MRI should be obtained, although these studies can be quite difficult to interpret in the immediate postpartum period.

15
CHAPTER

Circumcision

INDICATIONS AND CONTRAINDICATIONS

There is no true medical indication for a circumcision, because there is no clearly established health benefit from the procedure. Parents will request a circumcision for a variety of social and religious reasons. Most commonly, if the father has been circumcised, the parents will request that their boy also have his foreskin removed.

There are some contraindications to the procedure. Hypospadias, significant jaundice, or a bleeding disorder in the parents requires the obstetrician to reconsider the surgery and consult the pediatricians before proceeding.

INFORMED CONSENT

The degree of formal consent obtained before this brief, simple procedure varies among doctors. It is important to emphasize the optional nature of circumcision, particularly because some patients believe that the surgery is medically recommended.

ANESTHESIA

CONTROVERSY: Several studies have demonstrated the safety and efficacy of administering a local anesthetic in advance of circumcision. Whatever the evidence presented in JAMA, many doctors will no doubt view it as a waste of time with little benefit. Admittedly, it seems difficult sometimes to notice the difference, because many babies still cry quite vigorously, whether anesthetic is given or not.

The technique calls for injections of 0.2 to 0.4 mL of 1% lidocaine at the base of the penis at 2:00 and at 10:00, near the course of the two dorsal nerves of the penis. Prior to the injections, the skin at the base of the penis should be stabilized with gentle traction. Ideally, the needle should be advanced 2 to 5 mm through the skin in a posteromedial direction. Before administering the lidocaine, the syringe should be aspirated to be sure the needle is not intravascular. **PEARL: The lidocaine should be without epinephrine, and no more than 0.8 mL should be given.**

The practical result of these injections is that two small, practically contiguous blebs will form at the base of the penis. Anesthesia should be achieved within 2 to 3 minutes.

An alternative method is to place an anesthetic cream, a mixture of lidocaine 2.5% and prilocaine 2.5% (EMLA cream), on the penis 1 to 2 hours prior to the procedure.

PROCEDURE

The circumcision takes only 5 to 10 minutes, but like the episiotomy, it is not as easy as it first looks. Several techniques are available. The one described here uses the bell clamp, which comes in three sizes: 1.1, 1.3, and 1.5 (small, medium, and large).

1. Strap the baby into the specially designed tray. It is important to be sure the Velcro straps are attached above the knee to minimize the infant's kicking.
2. Put on your hat and mask, scrub, and put on gloves. The procedure is not as strictly sterile as an intra-abdominal operation.
3. Wash the penis with antiseptic and drape the area. Administer the lidocaine at this point if you plan to do so.
4. Grasp the foreskin at 11:00 and 1:00 with two hemostats. The urethral meatus is difficult to find, because the foreskin is somewhat folded over it. By grasping the foreskin in approximately the right location with hemostats and then applying gentle upward traction, you can confirm that you have appropriate placement of the hemostats.
5. Slide a closed hemostat oriented transversely just underneath the foreskin at 12:00. **PEARL: Be careful to keep the tips pointed outward, away from the penis itself.** Advance gently until resistance is encountered. Spread the tips, and withdraw slowly. This method serves to free up any loose adhesions between the foreskin and the glans penis. As the hemostat is being withdrawn, the glans can be visualized to confirm the anatomy. This step can be repeated several times until the foreskin slides more easily along the glans.
6. Clamp the foreskin with the hemostat at 12:00. The tips of the hemostat should be even with the bottom of the glans. Allow the clamp to remain on the skin for 30 seconds or so.
7. Cut along the foreskin at 12:00 with a scissors in the groove created by the clamp. The bleeding should be minimal, because the clamping step crushes the larger blood vessels.

8. With the help of the hemostats still affixed at 11:00 and 1:00, slide the foreskin back below the glans. This step further breaks up adhesions. I try to avoid the use of any instruments to break these attachments vigorously, because they can bleed, but gentle, blunt dissection is often necessary. In particular, the skin at 6:00 attaches relatively high on the glans. Do not mistake this for an adhesion, because this skin can bleed vigorously when disrupted.

9. Insert the appropriately sized bell under the foreskin and over the glans. It is helpful to use a third hemostat at 12:00 to pinch the foreskin together at the base of the bell to prevent it from sliding out.

10. Remove the hemostats at 11:00 and 1:00.

11. Take the flat base of the clamp and slide the bell portion through the hole at the end of the base. Gently affix the two prongs at the top of the bell protector to the receptacle on the clamp.

12. Look below the base of the clamp at the penis. The outline of the glans should be faintly discernible. Be sure that the skin here is not too taut or loose. Small adjustments in the amount of foreskin can be made at this point by gently pushing the tissue up or down through the loose clamp arrangement with 2 × 2 gauze.

13. Tighten the large nut at the end of the clamp. This method pulls the bell up against the clamp. This step is irreversible, because it crushes the blood vessels. It is important to be sure that the nut is turned as tightly as possible, because hemostasis depends on this step.

14. Some obstetricians like to wait for 5 minutes with the clamp on to be sure that hemostasis has been achieved, but 1 to 2 minutes may be all that is necessary. I use a knife blade without a handle to cut off the foreskin **distal** to

the clamp (above). It is important to get all the foreskin off and leave smooth edges. Otherwise the circumcision will leave a ragged edge of skin around the glans.

15. Loosen the clamp and gently slide the bell off the penis. Bleeding should be minimal. Should bleeding persist from specific arterioles, silver nitrate on a wooden applicator can be gently applied to the site for hemostasis.

16. Dress the wound with Vaseline and then dry gauze. Some hospitals have a policy that the baby is not discharged from the hospital until he urinates.

A FEW LAST WORDS

Over the years, I learned several important principles with regard to this surgery. **PEARL: First, you only have one chance to do it right.** Do not attempt to take off just a little bit more because this can be more difficult than it would appear. Second, it is sometimes difficult to tell how much is enough and not too much. As a rule, you want the skin of the penis to end at the glans. It rarely will. More commonly it will end a millimeter or so above or below the glans. Either case is an acceptable result. Finally, the penis can look amazingly bad the day after a properly performed procedure. It is typically black and blue and edematous.

4
PART

*Less Common
Problems*

16
CHAPTER

Hypertension in Pregnancy

The medical literature is filled with confusing and overlapping terminology describing hypertension in pregnancy. **PEARL: There are only two general types of hypertension in the obstetrical population: hypertension that was preexisting and hypertension that arises de novo during pregnancy. Pregnancy-induced hypertension (PIH) is the most inclusive word for the latter and includes the conditions known as preeclampsia and toxemia.** Eclampsia, in which seizures occur, and HELLP syndrome, in which thrombocytopenia and abnormal liver functions become manifest, are thought to represent clinical subsets of the condition known as PIH. To make matters more confusing, those with preexisting, chronic hypertension can develop PIH and indeed are more likely than their normotensive peers to do so.

PEARL: In previous years, edema was thought to be an important sign of PIH but this view has been rebuffed, because the majority of pregnant women experience at least some swelling by the end of pregnancy.

RISK FACTORS FOR PREGANCY-INDUCED HYPERTENSION

- First pregnancy
- Age greater than 40
- Multiple pregnancies
- Chronic hypertension

DEFINITIONS

Hypertension

The diagnosis of PIH is based on the finding of

- Diastolic pressure of 90 or above
- Systolic pressure of 140 or above

Proteinuria

PIH may be subclassified as *preeclampsia* if proteinuria (more than 300 mg in 24 hours) is present. As a practical rule, 2+ protein on a catheterized urinalysis is diagnostic of proteinuria in the absence of a urinary tract infection. A 2+ protein in the urine on a dipstick always raises a question about preeclampsia in a pregnant woman. This finding can also result from leaking amniotic fluid or an infection in the vagina or bladder, however, so it must always be checked using fresh, clean-catch urine or a catheterized specimen if the cause is not clear.

SEVERE PREGNANCY-INDUCED HYPERTENSION

Severe PIH can be quite a serious illness and is diagnosed when one of the following signs is present:

- Systolic pressure of 160 or more
- Diastolic pressure of 110 or more
- Oliguria (500 mL or less in 24 hours)
- Proteinuria of 5 g or more in 24 hours
- Neurological symptoms
    1. Headache or visual disturbances (severe)
    2. Seizures. Eclampsia is the occurrence of a seizure (not attributable to other causes) in a patient with PIH. Seizures can occur up to 1 week following delivery, but the period of highest risk ends after the first 24 hours following birth.

CONTROVERSY: Hyperreflexia used to be considered a sign of severe PIH, but the presence or absence of hyperreflexia is often hard to judge and does not contribute to the diagnosis of preeclampsia.

- Epigastric pain (can signal hepatic edema)
- Pulmonary edema or cyanosis
- Thrombocytopenia or hemolysis
- Intrauterine growth retardation (see Chapter 17)

LABORATORY EVIDENCE

Usually, patients with PIH show few laboratory abnormalities because most develop the illness close to term and do not become very ill. Tests for liver function, serum creatinine, CBC with platelets, and occasionally a D-dimer assay should be performed. For patients in labor, it is also prudent to send a type and screen in case cesarean section becomes necessary.

Things to look for include

- Increased (or even normal) hemoglobin. This factor can suggest hemoconcentration as vascular permeability increases and fluid begins to *third space*.

- Uric acid more than 5.5.
- Creatinine more than 1 (not completely reliable).
- BUN more than 10 (not completely reliable).
- Thrombocytopenia. Although disseminated intravascular coagulation (DIC) can occur in women with PIH, it is rather uncommon, particularly in the presence of a normal platelet count.

TREATMENT

PIH is cured with the delivery of the fetus and always worsens the longer the pregnancy continues. At term, the first principle of treatment is delivery. Before term is reached, the decision is more difficult because the fetus may also be in jeopardy from premature birth. **PEARL: PIH patients with severe disease are commonly delivered promptly at any gestational age.** Those women who only experience mild elevations in blood pressure and who have no stigmata of severe disease are usually managed as outpatients before term. Bed rest, frequent office visits, and assessments of fetal well-being such as ultrasound exams and nonstress tests are the mainstays of observation.

Seizure Prophylaxis

Begin with 4 to 6 g magnesium sulfate IV piggyback over 20 minutes and continue it at 2 g per hour. The therapeutic level is considered to be between 4 and 8 mEq/L.

CONTROVERSY: If deep tendon reflexes are brisk or clonus persists, the dose can be raised, usually in increments of 0.5 to 1 g/h.

Magnesium is cleared by the kidneys, and its level will climb with poor urine output. At levels of 10 to 12 mEq and above, muscle weakness, respiratory paralysis, and cardiac depression can ensue. **PEARL: Calcium gluconate should be administered IV in the event of magnesium toxicity.** Seizures can occur even with so-called therapeutic levels of magnesium.

To decrease significantly the level of magnesium in the bloodstream, it is more effective to stop the drug for 1 to 2 hours rather than simply to turn the infusion down. Similarly, repeated boluses (2 g over 10 minutes) can be given to raise the level, along with increasing the steady infusion rate.

The magnesium infusion is usually stopped 24 hours postpartum. While the magnesium infusion is continued, respirations and urine output are checked every hour (this procedure requires a Foley catheter). Deep tendon reflexes can serve as a rough guide to magnesium levels. A magnesium level should be checked when the deep tendon reflexes are significantly decreased, the respiratory rate decreases to 12 breaths per minute or less, or the urine output falls below 30 mL/h.

Ordering a so-called toxemia protocol in most hospitals is sufficient to indicate the need for hourly observation. Magnesium has killed hospitalized patients in the past through overdosage leading to respiratory depression. This fatal problem can occur if the magnesium infusion runs in wide open without an infusion pump.

In rabbits, magnesium can lower the diastolic blood pressure by as much as 10 mm Hg. In humans, this effect is less clear. **PEARL: If magnesium does have a beneficial impact on blood pressure, it is a small one.**

Magnesium can cause a modest decrease in fetal heart rate variability. It is important to remember that fetuses in mothers with PIH are in some jeopardy in the first place and their tracings have to be reviewed carefully.

Blood Pressure Control

When the diastolic blood pressure climbs to 110 or above, the possibility of intracerebral hemorrhage increases, and medication is indicated. Hydralazine (Apresoline), 5 to 10 mg IV push, is the drug of choice. The onset of effect occurs within 10 to 20 minutes, and the maximum effect is established at 20 to 40 minutes. If no response is seen in 15 minutes or so, the dose can be repeated. If three doses per hour are needed to keep the diastolic pressure under 110, an Apresoline drip beginning at 1 mg/h can be initiated. It is critical not to lower the blood pressure too precipitously, because this event can be harmful to both mother and fetus. Diastolic blood pressures under 105 usually are not treated. An alternative drug is labetalol, given 20 mg IV. The dose can be repeated at 10-minute intervals up to a total of 300 mg.

Oliguria

Oliguria is often the most vexing problem in those with severe disease, because there is no clearly preferable course of treatment. The patient is already predisposed to pulmonary edema and is very sensitive to fluid challenges. Paradoxically, the patient is also intravascularly volume depleted.

As a rule, patients with oliguria intrapartum warrant a central line to aid fluid replacement. A Swan-Ganz catheter is preferable, because there can be significant right-to-left cardiac dysfunction.

CONTROVERSY: Preeclamptic patients have an excess of total body sodium but are intravascularly depleted. Thus, some obstetricians argue for replacement with 0.2 normal saline (NS), whereas others insist on 0.9 NS.

In the United States, the use of Lasix to maintain urine output is discouraged, although in Britain, it is quite commonly used. Again, central line monitoring can be quite helpful in guiding therapy.

17
CHAPTER

Twins

INCIDENCE AND CAUSE

In a discussion of twins, a distinction should be made from the outset between monozygotic and dizygotic siblings. **PEARL: The frequency of monozygotic (identical) twinning is constant throughout the world and occurs at the rate of approximately 4 per 1000 pregnancies. In contrast, dizygotic (fraternal) twins occur at variable rates:**

Asians	2/1000 pregnancies
White Americans	6/1000
Black Americans	10/1000
Blacks (Nigeria)	40/1000

As can be seen, this highly variable dizygotic twinning rate influences the percentage of monozygotic twins born within a given population. For instance, two thirds of Asian twins are identical, whereas only 1 of every 10 twins born in Nigeria is monozygotic.

The differing epidemiology between the two types of twins suggests a different cause as well. Although the cause of embryo cleavage within 14 days of conception is poorly understood, identical twinning tends to be a randomly occurring event that is independent of family history and other factors. In sharp contrast, dizygotic twinning is related directly to the average circulating levels of the gonadotropins (particularly follicle-stimulating hormone [FSH]) in a given population. As a result, it occurs slightly more frequently in women as they age or when they undergo ovulation induction. It seems that serum FSH levels do vary among different ethnic groups: blacks have a higher level than whites, who, in turn, have a higher average serum FSH than Asians. The more FSH, the greater the probability of double ovulation in any given cycle.

DIAGNOSIS

There are three common ways to diagnose twins: physical exam, ultrasound, and maternal serum alpha-fetoprotein levels. Physical exam alone will fail to diagnose approximately 50% of twins. Although it may sound strange, in the days before ultrasound exams, obstetricians occasionally diagnosed twins by reaching inside the uterus to check on the placenta, only to have it kick them. A surprise indeed!

Although ultrasound is not completely accurate in diagnosing twins, its sensitivity is probably close to 99%—that is, of every 100 twin pregnancies, it will fail to diagnose 1. Therefore, ultrasound will miss one set of twins in roughly every 10,000 pregnant Americans.

In a roundabout way, even maternal serum alpha-fetoprotein can aid in the diagnosis of twins. Although it is primarily a screening tool for fetuses with neural tube defects, one cause of elevated levels (higher than 2.5 multiples of the median) can be twins. Part of the work-up of an initially elevated level is an ultrasound just for this purpose.

DIAGNOSIS OF ZYGOSITY

Determining the kinship between twins is often more than a matter of mere curiosity; it can have medical implications before and after birth. The first method that should be used is careful microscopic evaluation of the common membrane separating the pregnancies, using the following rules:

1. The thicker, outer membrane is the chorion, whereas the thinner membrane is the amnion.
2. **PEARL: Monochorionic twins are always monozygotic.** They can either share amnionic membranes or have separate ones. Twins that share one amnion, while uncommon, are at extreme risk for cord accidents, and dual survival of monoamnionic twins is rare indeed. The identification of some membrane separating the fetuses during ultrasound is of more than just passing interest.
3. Dichorionic twins are usually, but **not** always, dizygotic. Identical twins occasionally have separate chorions.

Thus, most identical twins can be diagnosed with certainty on the basis of the placenta, but the relationship between fraternal, same-sex twins cannot be proven similarly.

Two other techniques are commonly used to classify same-sex twins. The first is genetic blood typing, in which a minimum number of proteins (usually eight) on red blood cells are compared. If all eight proteins are identical, the probability of monozygosity is more than 95% (depending on the specific proteins). Of course, this probability rises with the number of proteins that are found to be shared between the siblings (as long as there are no differences).

A much cheaper method is to wait until the siblings are in their early teens and then ask their parents, "Are they as alike as two peas in a pod?" If both answer yes, the probability of monozygosity is greater than 90%.

MORBIDITY AND MORTALITY

The prenatal care for women with twin gestations differs somewhat from the standard protocol for those with singleton pregnancies. This is chiefly due to the fact that the perinatal mortality rate is four times higher than the singleton rate for the first twin and five times higher for the second twin. It is worthwhile to review briefly the causes for some of these adverse outcomes, because much of prenatal care is directed at averting them.

Prematurity

Approximately 50% of twin gestations deliver by 37 weeks. **PEARL: Prematurity is the biggest single factor in the high twin neonatal mortality rate and is a contributing factor in the majority of these deaths.**

Intrauterine Growth Retardation

Definition

Another risk of multiple gestation is intrauterine growth retardation (IUGR).

CONTROVERSY: IUGR is a difficult term to define. A better word for this idea is malnourished *fetus. This concept refers to the observation that some fetuses appear malnourished when born thin and underweight for their length and gestational age. These infants are usually easy to identify on visual inspection after birth, but many authors have difficulty defining the term precisely. Probably the most widely used definition is a baby weighing under 2500 g who is also in the lowest 10th percentile weight group for his or her gestational age. Of course, this definition suggests that infants weighing over 2500 g cannot be classified as* growth retarded, *yet some of them clearly appear to be malnourished.*

Diagnosis

The antenatal diagnosis rests chiefly on ultrasound. With this technique, two types of IUGR are identifiable: symmetrical and asymmetrical. Symmetrical IUGR (the more severe form) occurs when both the body and the head have poor growth over serial scans. **PEARL: Asymmetrical IUGR (the more common variety) may occur in mild cases of malnourishment, because the head continues to grow at a more or less normal rate while the body has poor growth.**

The ultrasound standards used for judging growth rate depend on the gestational age and the population studied. Biparietal diameters (width of the fetal head) and abdominal circumferences are most used to judge fetal growth, although other measurements such as head circumference and femur length also may be of interest. There is debate about whether singleton growth curves and measurements can be appropriately applied to twins. Below-average volumes of amniotic fluid are also highly suggestive of IUGR, although the mechanism is unclear.

Discordant twins are a special situation unique

to multiple gestation. **PEARL: There is no standard definition of discordant twins, but a commonly used criterion is a 25% difference in birth weight.** Significant differences in growth within twin pairs can significantly increase the perinatal mortality rate, particularly for the smaller twin. The best way to follow discordant growth is with serial ultrasound exams, but there are few data regarding criteria for intervention.

Treatment of IUGR is difficult at best. Bed rest, smoking cessation, and attention to maternal nutrition may be of modest benefit. Nonstress tests may be used in an effort to identify those malnourished fetuses at particular risk of demise. In extreme cases, premature delivery may be considered.

Risks

The diagnosis of IUGR carries with it an increased probability of short-term and long-term problems. As IUGR fetuses often have reduced amounts of amniotic fluid and relatively thin umbilical cords, the chances of compromise during labor are higher. Immediately after birth, hypothermia and hypoglycemia may emerge as problems owing to decreased liver glycogen stores. Over the long term, these initially malnourished babies are thought to be prone to developmental delays and impaired school performance.

Twin-Twin Transfusion Syndrome

Peculiar to monozygotic twins, this problem occurs when the placental arteries of one twin empty into the veins of the other. As a result, one twin becomes polycythemic, while the other becomes anemic. This potentially fatal problem can sometimes be diagnosed by ultrasound.

Additional Problems

Risks for the mother include an increased likelihood of hyperemesis gravidarum (severe nausea and vomiting), PIH, and postpartum hemorrhage (from uterine atony). Iron deficiency anemia is also more likely in mothers of twins. Other risks for the fetuses include an increased probability of congenital anomalies and malpresentation during labor.

PRENATAL CARE

Although recommendations vary greatly among obstetricians, an example of a prenatal treatment plan is the following:

1. Weekly or biweekly prenatal visits after 24 weeks to check blood pressure and cervical dilatation
2. Monthly ultrasound exams to measure growth in the late second trimester and beyond
3. Markedly decreased activity or bed rest in the third trimester
4. Weekly nonstress testing at 34 to 36 weeks through delivery (earlier if IUGR is suspected)

These steps are designed to detect and avert the two largest threats to a twin gestation—prematurity and poor growth.

LABOR AND DELIVERY

The two chief areas of controversy in the delivery of twins are when to do a cesarean section for malpresentation and how to manage the delivery of the second twin if the first is delivered vaginally. It should be emphasized that there are several legitimate approaches.

Because twins are almost invariably smaller at a given gestation, there is less concern about breech fetuses becoming entrapped within the maternal bony pelvis. However, premature breeches may still be better off with cesarean birth (see Chapter 18). One concern about delivering the first twin as a breech if the second twin is vertex is that, rarely, the chin of the first may lock with the chin of the second, impeding delivery. **PEARL: If the first fetus presents head first, there is less concern about delivering the subsequent baby as a breech vaginally.** Gestational age is also an important issue in deciding the route of delivery, because very premature fetuses may experience more difficulties during labor. As a practical matter, many obstetricians will order an abdominal x-ray or an ultrasound at the outset of labor to identify more clearly the presentations and relative positioning of the twins.

With regard to delivery of the second twin, it was certainly true that in decades past, morbidity and mortality rose with an increasing time interval between births. The mean time interval between deliveries is 20 minutes or so. With the advent of electronic fetal monitoring, intervention at some arbitrary time limit seems less necessary. Because the condition of the second twin can deteriorate rapidly, however, emergency cesarean section occasionally becomes necessary. Many obstetricians try to leave the membranes intact around the second twin for as long as possible to reduce the chance of cord prolapse.

An alternative to cesarean section for rapid delivery of a breech second twin is a procedure known as *breech extraction*, in which the feet of the fetus are grasped and brought out through the vagina. If the amnionic membranes are not ruptured by this time, most obstetricians prefer to leave them intact during a breech extraction. Breech extractions are often done under halothane anesthesia to permit uterine relaxation.

After both infants are born, uterine atony is the largest concern before and after delivery of the placenta. If bleeding is unusually brisk, the placentas can be removed manually. For heavy bleeding after the placentas have been delivered, bimanual uterine massage is usually immediately effective in helping the uterus contract. Of course, oxytocin and methylergonovine (Methergine) may also be beneficial.

18

Breech

DEFINITION

Two sets of definitions are commonly encountered in any discussion of breeches—those referring to presentation and those referring to delivery.

Presentation

- **Frank breech.** The presenting part of the fetus is the buttocks, and the legs are both flexed and parallel to the thorax (Fig. 18–1A).
- **Complete breech.** The fetus has assumed a sitting position within the birth canal, but the buttocks are still the presenting part (Fig. 18–1B).
- **Footling breech.** One or both feet are now inferior to the buttocks and will be the first part to deliver (Fig. 18–1C). This category is further divided into single-footling breech and double-footling breech.

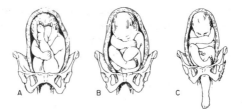

Figure 18–1. Breech presentations. **A,** Frank breech presentation. **B,** Complete breech presentation. **C,** Footling breech presentation. (From Bonica, JJ: Principles and Practice of Obstetric Analgesia and Anesthesia. FA Davis, Philadelphia, 1967, p 1223, with permission.)

Delivery

- **Spontaneous breech.** The fetus is delivered without any assistance other than support of the body as it emerges.
- **Assisted breech or partial breech extraction.** The fetal arms and head are manipulated after delivery of the umbilicus. This route of delivery also describes the use of forceps for the head, although the use of forceps is often specifically mentioned in any description of the birth.
- **Breech extraction.** This method of delivery involves grasping both feet and pulling the fetus through and out of the vagina. This is rarely done except possibly for rapid delivery of the second twin.

INCIDENCE AND CAUSE

PEARL: At term, 3% to 4% of fetuses present as breeches. Of all breeches, 65% are frank, versus 25% for footling and 10% for complete breech.

Gestational age has a significant impact on the probability of breech presentation. In the mid-second trimester, roughly one-fourth of fetuses are breech, whereas at 28 to 30 weeks, only 8% present in this way. The percentage declines further as term approaches.

Why are some babies breech? No one really knows for sure. Theories include fundal implantation of the placenta (which only occurs in 7% of pregnancies) and some abnormality of fetal muscle tone. Some investigators have found motor abnormalities in children who were breech regardless of route of delivery. They speculate that the fetus was breech because of impaired ability to move within the uterus.

RISKS

Fetuses that are breech are exposed to greater risks during labor and delivery than those who emerge head first. **PEARL: The risks stem largely from two main problems: head entrapment and cord prolapse.**

Head Entrapment

When a vertex fetus is too large for the maternal pelvis, progress in labor will ultimately stop. Whether delivery by cesarean is accomplished in minutes or in hours, the fetal condition does not usually change significantly without other complicating factors. The key difference in the delivery of a breech is that the largest part of the body, the head, is the last to deliver. Occasionally, the smaller thorax will deliver when the head will not. In such a circumstance, completing the delivery of the infant can be quite a challenge, as cesarean at this point is not usually a viable option (as the infant would literally have to be put back into the vagina and uterus). Because the baby cannot breathe while its oropharynx is still in the vagina and the umbilical cord is now compromised, the obstetrician has minutes rather than hours to accomplish delivery. The frightening feature of head entrapment is that it can be unpredictable, just as it is difficult to know which fetus and mother will experience cephalopelvic disproportion without a trial of labor. It is thought that proper selection of mothers for labor with breech presentations will keep this risk to a minimum.

Umbilical Cord Prolapse

With frank breech or vertex presentations, this obstetrical emergency occurs only in roughly 5 per 1000 labors. This risk rises to 50 per 1000 with complete breeches and 100 per 1000 for footling breeches. As a result, most obstetricians will consider labor and vaginal birth only for frank breeches.

MANAGEMENT

Of all breech babies in the United States, 90% are delivered by cesarean section. With the well-recognized increased maternal morbidity and mortality rates for operative delivery, the key issue for breech delivery is, "Are there situations in which vaginal delivery poses no greater danger to the fetus than cesarean birth?" The literature suggests that there are indeed circumstances in which labor may be safely attempted, although there is still much controversy. Pragmatically, it is simply not possible to randomize 10,000 mothers with breech presentations and measure the outcome with different protocols.

Vaginal Birth

1. **Gestational age.** Contrary to intuition, small, premature fetuses may actually have a higher risk from vaginal birth than those who are larger. Because the head-to-abdomen ratio is larger in the first half of the third trimester than in the second half, soft tissue entrapment poses a real threat. Many obstetricians advocate cesarean delivery for even frank breeches when the fetus is less then 34 weeks.
2. **Frank breech.** Frank breeches seem most appropriate for vaginal birth because they do not have an increased risk of cord prolapse, as do complete and footling breeches.
3. **Estimated fetal weight.** Although neither ultrasound nor physical exam is entirely reliable, some suggest that an infant with a birth weight between 2500 and 3800 g has the least chance for morbidity from vaginal birth.
4. **Prior deliveries.** Some specialists advocate that primigravidas should not attempt labor with a breech, although the medical evidence supporting this contention is weak. This issue remains very controversial.
5. **Oxytocin stimulation.** Some obstetricians use oxytocin to stimulate or induce labor, but this approach, too, is controversial. Some argue that medical augmentation of labor may force a fetus with only a marginal fit through the pelvis. Of course, without oxytocin, some mothers

who might otherwise have had a vaginal birth will require cesarean section. This situation would include those who do not go into labor after premature rupture of membranes or those who require an induction of labor for medical reasons. Again, the view on oxytocin use during breech labor varies widely.

6. **X-ray pelvimetry.** Although it has largely been discredited for predicting cephalopelvic disproportion with vertex presentations, x-ray measurement of bony landmarks may have some merit in those with breech. It can be used to eliminate those women with unusually small dimensions from undergoing a trial of labor. As with other issues in breech delivery, there is little consensus on its usefulness.

7. **Head hyperextension.** A small number of breech infants (5%) will have a *hyperextended head*. This means that the head is flexed backward on the neck, which is also known as *stargazing*. This posture has been associated with increased probability of head entrapment or trauma to the cervical spine and is usually diagnosed by x-ray study.

8. **Cervical exam.** The lower the breech and the more dilated the cervix at the start of labor, the more favorable the prognosis. Various investigators have tried to establish guidelines, but there is no universal agreement.

9. **Progress in labor.** Any vaginal trial of labor for breech presupposes that the labor progresses smoothly and that there is steady cervical dilatation and descent of the presenting part. Of course, electronic fetal monitoring is of value in helping to ensure a favorable outcome.

The best candidates for labor are those who have spontaneous contractions with good cervical dilatation at the outset and medium-size babies. Ideally, the fetus should be a frank breech without head hyperextension. Because fetal posture is best demonstrated by x-ray study, and fetal weight is more accurately predicted by ultrasound, many obstetricians obtain both studies at the outset of labor. Many authorities claim that vaginal birth poses no increased risk to the fetus and increased safety to the mother in properly selected cases.

Cesarean Section

As mentioned previously, 90% of breeches are delivered by cesarean section. One unique consideration in the delivery of these infants is the orientation of the uterine incision. Hyperextension of the head and difficult delivery are still concerns if the uterine incision is too small. As a result, some specialists advocate a lower cervical vertical incision to ensure an atraumatic birth. A large enough transverse incision may often suffice.

External Version

External version entails manipulating the fetus through the maternal abdominal wall in an effort to turn it to the head first position. There are several supportive studies in the medical literature. In general, the problems include separation of the placenta from the uterus, uterine rupture, fetal-maternal hemorrhage, and failure. Failure comes in two forms: an inability to turn the baby at the outset and a subsequent return to the breech position after an initially successful version. In the debate on external version, the disagreement does not concern the existence or nature of the various risks but their probability.

For those patients who seem to be appropriate candidates for version, the procedure is generally done in the hospital at 36 to 38 weeks' gestation, with provisions made for immediate cesarean section. External version is not recommended for those already in labor. An IV is established, and an operating room is prepared. An ultrasound is used to guide the repositioning of the fetus, which is accomplished by steady, gentle hand-over-hand pressure. Agents that relax the uterus (such as ritodrine) are often administered before and during the procedure. Rh-negative mothers should probably receive Rh immune globulin.

19
CHAPTER

Preterm Labor

This chapter on preterm labor is meant to be only a thumbnail sketch of clinically relevant facts. Junior residents are encouraged to consult more experienced physicians whenever they deal with potential labor before term.

EPIDEMIOLOGY

Prematurity remains the leading cause of death for neonates without congenital anomalies. By definition, this is birth after 20 weeks' gestation and before 37 completed weeks (from the first day of the last menstrual period). In the United States, the incidence of preterm delivery is roughly 10%, and it is a factor in the majority of neonatal deaths.

Because a newborn's weight can be determined more accurately than his or her gestational age, birthweight has occasionally been used as a surrogate for the study of prematurity. Birthweight has been described as low (<2500 g), very low (<1500 g), or extemely low (<1000 g).

Some characteristics of a patient's history may predict an increased risk for preterm labor. Unfortunately, such historical factors do not permit a very sensitive or specific forecast for prematurity. Examples of factors associated with subsequent early labor include a history of preterm labor in a prior pregnancy, smoking more than half a pack a day, diethylstilbestrol (DES) exposure in utero, some uterine anomalies such as bicornuate uterus, and history of a cone biopsy (removal of the central portion of the cervix to detect premalignant and malignant conditions). Certain complications of pregnancy have also been thought to increase the risk of preterm labor. These include pyelonephritis, advanced cervical dilatation, excess amniotic fluid, and of course, twins.

DIAGNOSIS

PEARL: The diagnosis of preterm labor rests heavily on its definition: uterine contractions leading to progressive cervical dilatation and effacement before 37 completed weeks of pregnancy. Although the definition seems clear enough, there are certain practical difficulties in making this diagnosis. First, the early contractions of preterm labor may not be as distinct to the patient as active labor at term. Many will describe their contractions as "the baby balling up," back pain, or intestinal cramping. Indeed, some patients may have diarrhea at the time they begin their labor, so that their presentation may be quite confused.

Because the success of intervention steadily declines with advancing dilatation, there is some pressure on the physician to decide rapidly. On the other hand, because the intervention often includes strict bed rest for the rest of pregnancy and a complete cessation of work, the obstetrician is also inclined to avoid overdiagnosing the condition. Finally, there are some patients who will have regular contractions for a few hours at a time or even days who do not have cervical change and who will ultimately deliver at term. Although a minority, this group of women further complicates making an accurate diagnosis.

The differential diagnosis of preterm labor includes disorders of the uterus, bowel, urinary tract, and even the abdominal musculature. Separation of the placenta from the uterus can indeed cause contractions and even labor, but this condition should be considered as a separate entity because it can cause immediate fetal and even maternal death (see Chapter 20). Other disorders of the uterus that can be confused with preterm labor include the pain of degenerating fibroids and, rarely, fetal movement.

Intestinal disorders, including appendicitis, spastic bowel, and constipation, can mimic early preterm labor. Indeed, the uterus may actually contract occasionally in response to these disorders, but premature delivery is not a common outcome.

Cystitis, pyelonephritis, and ureteral stones can all mimic the symptoms of preterm labor. As with the bowel disorders, these conditions can actually be associated with uterine contractions, and pyelonephritis is thought to be a risk factor for preterm delivery. Finally, some patients present with episodic lower abdominal pain that proves to be a result of some strain within or trauma to the abdominal wall.

In practice, any change in cervical dilatation or effacement in the presence of uterine contractions may be considered evidence of labor before term. Patients who present before 37 completed weeks with contractions and who are 2 cm or more dilated or more than 80% effaced are highly likely to be in labor. **PEARL: It is not unusual for multiparous patients to be 2 cm dilated in the middle of the third trimester, but those with contractions should usually**

be treated. Finally, regular contractions (eight or so in an hour) in the presence of ruptured membranes may also be regarded as labor, although the management may be different than when the membranes are intact.

Two diagnostic tests have been developed in an effort to identify those at high risk for preterm labor. Fetal fibronectin is a glycoprotein found in cervical secretions, which increases during early labor.

CONTROVERSY: The role, if any, of fetal fibronectin testing is still being defined, but it seems that a negative test result is more predictive of the lack of imminent labor than a positive test result is of early labor.

The second diagnostic test is daily home contraction monitoring via telemetry.

CONTROVERSY: The general consensus in the medical literature is that monitoring contractions by telemetry is not effective in prolonging pregnancies or improving neonatal outcome.

TREATMENT

PEARL: No treatment to date has been proven to be very effective in delaying delivery for more than a day or two. Remarkably, virtually all of the pharmaceutical agents used to treat preterm labor can have significant side effects or risks for mother, fetus, or both. This lack of efficacy is easily explained by the fact that the biochemistry of labor remains elusive, and therefore a precise scientific approach to treatment remains in the future.

Many obstetrical personnel, particularly maternity nurses, have high expectations for treatment based on experience. Paradoxically, because treatment has so little effect, if any, many patients receive medication at the earliest sign of preterm labor. Because many, if not the majority, of them are not destined to deliver in any case, this practice tends to create a spurious impression of the efficacy of treatment.

As it stands now, treatment consists primarily of two modalities: bed rest and medication.

Bed Rest

A variety of studies suggest that bed rest is beneficial in either forestalling labor or helping interrupt established labor in association with medication. Because none of these studies are prospective randomized trials and many of them pertain to twins, the precise efficacy of bed rest is still uncertain. Nevertheless, virtually all obstetricians will incorporate rigorous bed rest in the long-term treatment of anyone with preterm labor.

Pharmacological Agents

IV hydration is often recommended as an early form of intervention, prior to initiating pharmacological agents. Although I have seen many apparent successes with hydration alone, it may be that uterine activity ceases with the passage of a few hours rather than through volume expansion. **PEARL: Two main classes of drugs are used to treat uterine contractions: beta sympathomimetics and magnesium.** Other agents, such as ethanol and prostaglandin inhibitors, may have some benefit in inhibiting labor but are not as widely used. Ethanol has very unpleasant side effects, and the prostaglandin inhibitors simply have not been studied as much. There are also lingering concerns about their safety for the fetus.

Beta Sympathomimetics

So named because they preferentially stimulate the beta-adrenergic receptors, the two drugs most commonly used are ritodrine (Yutopar) and terbutaline. Terbutaline is not approved by the Food and Drug Administration (FDA) specifically for the treatment of preterm labor, but it is very similar to ritodrine in its physiological effects and has been used as an alternative. Terbutaline can be given intravenously, orally, or even as a subcutaneous injection. Its chief advantage over ritodrine is its substantially lower cost.

These agents are preferred because they show some predilection for beta$_2$ receptor activity (myometrium, bronchioles, and blood vessels) versus beta$_1$ receptor activity (myocardium, intestinal tract). The beta$_2$ responses include decreased smooth muscle tone in the uterus, bronchioles, and vasculature. Urinary output is also decreased, and both glycogenolysis and insulin release are increased. Because these drugs do have some beta$_1$ activity, they will also increase pulse rate. Pulmonary edema has been reported in patients taking beta sympathomimetics. However, pulmonary edema is an uncommon complication, and it seems unpredictable and is not necessarily related to dosage.

The side effects of beta sympathomimetics can be predicted from their physiological action. **PEARL: Decreased diastolic blood pressure (and faintness or dizziness), pounding and rapid heart rate, and an increase in serum glucose with a corresponding decrease in potassium are all prominent features of treatment with beta sympathomimetics. In addition, many patients will actually develop a tremor or jitteriness.** The net result is that some patients may become quite uncomfortable at the higher doses of medication.

There are no known long-term ill effects from intrauterine exposure to beta sympathomimetics. The drugs do cause an increase in the fetal heart rate. As might be expected, neonates exposed to these agents during labor have temporary hypoglycemia, neonatal ileus, and hypotension.

Sample Ritodrine Protocol

1. Establish that preterm labor is occurring, and obtain maternal medical history. Magnesium (discussed later) may be a better choice in the event of maternal diabetes, bleeding, or heart condition.
2. Obtain CBC with platelets, and serum electrolytes and glucose. A pretreatment ECG may be warranted to help evaluate any subsequent chest pain or cardiac irregularities. Fluid balance should be carefully monitored. Occasionally a Foley catheter is of benefit.
3. Begin an IV drip, and then start the medication at 50 to 100 µg/min. A computerized infusion pump should be used.
4. Increase the dose by 50 µg/min every 15 minutes until contractions are fewer than four per hour or to a maximum dose of 350 µg/min.
5. Output and vitals should be checked frequently. In particular, once a maternal pulse of 140 is achieved, it is wise not to increase the dose further, regardless of the success of labor inhibition.
6. Maintain steady-state dosing for 6 to 12 hours. As a rule, fetal monitoring is continuous, and the patient remains observed in labor and delivery until she is stable on oral medication.
7. Wean to oral medication by giving 10 to 20 mg of ritodrine orally 1 hour prior to stopping the IV medication. Follow up with 10 to 20 mg of oral ritodrine every 2 to 4 hours as necessary.

The oral dosing is determined empirically by observing the patient in the hospital for at least 1 or 2 days.

8. Hypokalemia and elevated glucoses while the patient is receiving therapy are not treated unless they represent preexisting conditions or are abnormal in the extreme.

Magnesium Sulfate

The mechanism of action of magnesium is thought to be related to calcium antagonism. That is, it seems that magnesium decreases the intracellular free calcium necessary for smooth muscle contraction. Unfortunately, magnesium has this effect on all muscle. At 4 mEq/mL, deep tendon reflexes tend to be decreased, whereas at levels of 12 mEq/mL, respiratory depression occurs, as well as cardiac impairment. At intermediate levels, patients may experience flushing, headaches, and nystagmus. In practice, one of the most debilitating side effects is a difficult-to-describe dysphoria in which many feel as though they are trapped within a dark cloud.

As with the beta sympathomimetics, there are no known ill long-term effects of magnesium on the fetus. Occasionally, a decrease in muscle tone may be noted initially if the neonate was born while the mother was being treated with large doses of magnesium, as it crosses the placenta.

Sample Magnesium Protocol

1. Follow steps 1 and 2 in the preceding ritodrine protocol. An ECG is less necessary for those given magnesium, although it might be helpful to confirm a normal calcium level before starting the drug. As with ritodrine, urine output should be watched closely, because magnesium levels can rise in the presence of oliguria.

2. Give a loading dose of 4 g over 10 to 20 minutes

and then infuse magnesium at the rate of 1 to 3 g/h. A computerized infusion pump should be used. The dosage of magnesium should not exceed 4 g/h because toxic levels may be reached.

3. Increase the dose in ½-g quantities every 15 minutes until the contractions are four or fewer per hour.

4. The dose should probably not be increased in the presence of significant nystagmus. If the respiratory rate slows on magnesium, stop the drug at least temporarily.

5. There is debate about the usefulness of checking magnesium levels, because the clinical status of the patient usually is a reasonably reliable indicator of drug level. Nevertheless, it is not unreasonable to check the serum magnesium every 6 to 12 hours. Keep in mind that it takes hours for magnesium to equilibrate in the bloodstream. Both respiratory rate and deep tendon reflexes should be carefully monitored, although the deep tendon reflexes are more sensitive.

6. After uterine relaxation has been achieved, some obstetricians switch to oral beta sympathomimetics. There have been reports of oral magnesium supplementation, but this approach requires very large quantities of medicine to achieve significant blood levels.

Contraindications to Tocolysis

Under some conditions, the risk to the fetus and to the mother is less with a preterm birth than with tocolysis. For example, with extreme maternal hemorrhage, it is probably more prudent to accomplish delivery rather than to delay it. Using tocolytics in women with ruptured membranes remains controversial and seems to be less effective.

Follow-up

Patients at high risk for preterm labor or already receiving medication for it are usually placed on complete bed rest at home.

CONTROVERSY: There is some thought that sexual intercourse may hasten labor as a result of the prostaglandins in semen. The notion that orgasm may precipitate labor has not been confirmed in the medical literature.

Patients are advised to have weekly office visits, during which the cervix is checked. Those who have changed from one week to the next can be monitored for several hours (usually in labor and delivery) to be sure that they are not actively contracting. Tocolytic agents can be stopped at the beginning of the 37th week.

PROGRESSION OF PRETERM LABOR

Once labor is well established, tocolysis usually fails. Specifically, few patients who dilate to 4 cm or beyond with documentable contractions will to respond to intervention. If delivery appears inevitable, the medications should be stopped and the pediatricians should be notified. The time course of preterm labor is notoriously variable, and the cervix does not need to dilate as completely to permit the passage of a premature fetus. Keep in mind that there is an increased incidence of breech before term and that the very low birth weight breech fetuses may be better off with cesarean delivery.

THE NEWBORN
PREMATURE INFANT

Morbidity and Mortality

The probability of survival for a given neonate depends on both its gestational age and birth weight. A newborn at 26 weeks who weighs 900 g is more likely to survive than one who weighs 700 g. Conversely, the 700-g fetus who is actually 28 weeks' gestational age has a better prognosis than one at 26 weeks' gestational age with the same weight.

Assuming an average weight, the approximate probability of survival at 26 weeks is on the order of 30%. At 29 weeks, more than 90% of those delivered will live. These statistics have been improving steadily over the last decade.

Of course, another issue is the quality of life for survivors. This remains somewhat controversial. As gestational age increases, the long-term deficits among survivors markedly decrease. Most of those delivered at and beyond 29 weeks are not handicapped, and even most delivered before, who survive, this time will grow to lead normal lives.

By and large, there are at least six major threats to the premature neonate:

1. **Respiratory distress.** This problem is discussed later.
2. **Patent ductus arteriosus.** Particularly in very premature infants, the ductus arteriosus may fail to close promptly, resulting in at least a temporary left-to-right shunt that can result in congestive heart failure. In extreme cases, prostaglandin inhibitors or surgical ligature may be necessary.
3. **Intraventricular hemorrhage and neurological deficits.** The cerebral blood vessels seem

particularly fragile in premature infants. The veins are prone to tears, which can lead to significant intracranial hemorrhage. In more severe cases, the blood can leak into the ventricles, which may interfere with absorption of intraventricular fluid and further compromise neural tissue. *Traumatic birth* has traditionally been thought to be a cause, but it is becoming increasingly evident that preterm fetuses are prone to this problem no matter what the route of delivery. There is an association between prematurity, low birth weight, and cerebral palsy, but the etiology is unclear.

4. **Hyperbilirubinemia.** Hyperbilirubinemia may become a problem in preterm infants because the liver may not have matured enough to fully metabolize bilirubin in the first few days of life. With high enough levels sustained over a period of time, bilirubin toxicity can occur, causing brain damage. In mild to moderate elevations of bilirubin, exposure of the newborn to ultraviolet light assists the metabolism of bilirubin. In more severe cases, exchange transfusions may be required, in which the neonate's blood is removed and replaced with donor blood with a low bilirubin content.

5. **Sepsis.** Premature infants are less able to fend off bacteria and can succumb rapidly to infections that full-term infants would normally survive. Diagnosing sepsis in these infants can also be quite difficult, because they show few signs or symptoms of illness until the infection is quite advanced. Pneumonia and meningitis are infections of particular concern.

6. **Feeding difficulties.** As can be imagined, nutrition of the premature infant is no simple matter. Not only are his or her nutritional requirements not fully known, but also the gastrointestinal tract is frequently not prepared to be the primary source of nutrient processing.

As an example, coordination between swallowing and respiration does not reliably occur before 32 to 34 weeks, and aspiration of oral intake is a problem before this time. Frequently, gavage feeding (through a tube that passes through the mouth or nose into the stomach) is necessary. In extremely ill neonates, hyperalimentation may be required.

Respiratory Distress Syndrome

One of the biggest problems facing the premature infant is respiration. The major obstacle to sustained spontaneous respiration is the absence of surfactant, a lipoprotein mixture that decreases the surface tension within the lungs. Without surfactant, the lungs are relatively stiff and inflexible, leading to rapid tiring of the newborn. Without mechanical assistance, many would succumb.

At 34 to 36 weeks, most fetuses begin producing surfactant in significant quantities. The probability of respiratory distress syndrome (RDS) can be predicted while the fetus is still in utero from measuring lipoproteins within the amnionic fluid (through amniocentesis). By measuring the ratio of phosphatidylcholine (lecithin) to sphingomyelin (the L/S ratio), the likelihood of RDS can be estimated. Among those with an L/S of 2:1 or more, RDS occurs less than 2% of the time. Those with a ratio of less than 2:1 have up to a 50% chance of developing the disease. As a practical matter, the L/S ratio can help obstetricians decide whether or not to use drugs to inhibit labor. For instance, in a pregnant woman at 35 weeks who is contracting, a rapidly obtained L/S ratio can serve as a guide to how vigorous an effort should be made to stop labor. Other tests, some of which can be performed quite rapidly with automated equipment, have been developed to aid in determining fetal lung maturity.

Another issue encountered in obstetrics is the

use of glucocorticoids to enhance fetal lung maturity. There is some evidence that steroids given 2 to 7 days in advance of delivery between 24 and 34 weeks' gestation may promote surfactant production. **PEARL: In 1995, a National Institutes of Health (NIH) consensus panel recommended steroid administration to pregnant women at less than 34 weeks' gestation in whom delivery was believed to be likely within the next week.** A commonly used regimen is dexamethasone 5 mg intramuscularly every 12 hours for up to four doses.

CONTROVERSY: The presence of ruptured membranes, maternal diabetes, hypertension, multiple gestation, and intrauterine growth retardation makes the benefits of steroid treatment less clear. There are no known short-term or long-term ill effects on the fetus, although paradoxically there is some evidence that steroids may induce labor. Also, the risk of pulmonary edema in patients being treated with beta sympathomimetics may be increased with the concomitant use of glucocorticoids.

Exogenously introduced surfactant became widely available in the early 1990s. Available in an aerosol spray, it is dispersed throughout the lungs via intubation and mechanical ventilation. **PEARL: Artificial surfactant has revolutionized care in the neonatal intensive care unit and has made RDS much less common.** It can be used as either prophylaxis or treatment for RDS.

PRETERM PREMATURE RUPTURE OF THE MEMBRANES

Premature rupture of membranes (PROM) refers to the amnionic membranes breaking before the onset of labor, whether at term or before. Of course, preterm PROM occurs before 37 completed weeks' gestation. Preterm PROM occurs in roughly 1% of pregnancies.

Complications

The two chief complications of preterm PROM are labor and uterine infection. **PEARL: About 80% of pregnant patients will spontaneously go into labor within 1 week of membrane rupture.** Of course, the vast majority will be destined to delivery prematurely. Because many of these patients will spontaneously dilate and efface in the apparent absence of contractions, the diagnosis of labor can be quite difficult to make.

Infection is perhaps even more of a concern, because it can definitely jeopardize maternal well-being. Those who develop a uterine infection while the fetus remains inside (chorioamnionitis) can become septic and deteriorate quite rapidly, although this is not often the case. The signs and symptoms of chorioamnionitis include an elevated maternal temperature (any reading over 99.4°F should be regarded suspiciously), fetal or maternal tachycardia, and uterine contractions or tenderness.

Known chorioamnionitis is a contraindication to tocolysis. Prolonging the pregnancy under these circumstances increases both maternal and fetal risk, at least in extreme cases. Fortunately, tocolysis is rarely successful in those with chorioamnionitis. When it is difficult to distinguish between labor and infection, some obstetricians use magnesium to stall for time until the diagnosis becomes clearer. Ritodrine, which raises both the maternal and fetal pulse, can cloud the issue.

Many advocate obtaining serial white blood cell counts to assist in detection of chorioamnionitis. Although this is not a bad idea, a significantly elevated white count is usually a late finding. Maternal pulse and temperature seem to be more sensitive.

Diagnosis and Management

In the initial assessment of preterm PROM, several steps should be taken immediately. First, the diagnosis should be confirmed by sterile speculum exam, nitrazine paper, and the finding of a ferning pattern of the fluid as it dries under magnification. **PEARL: If PROM is either confirmed or suspected, a digital cervical exam should be avoided unless delivery is imminent (within hours), because this practice has been linked to an increased probability of chorioamnionitis.**

Fluid should be collected for surfactant studies, although this is not always possible. Fluid is collected by attaching the plastic tube from an IV starter set (without the steel introducer) to the end of a 5-mL syringe and depositing the fluid in a plain glass test tube. (A larger syringe often will not pass though the opening of the speculum.) The fluid should be obtained from the posterior vault, taking care to avoid the mucus that is often present, which will clog the plastic tube.

Finally, cervical cultures for betahemolytic strep, gonorrhea, and chlamydia should be obtained, because the presence of these organisms is associated with increased neonatal morbidity. At the least, mothers with preterm PROM should be placed on bed rest.

CONTROVERSY: Some obstetricians will have the patient observed in the hospital for several days (if not longer), depending on the patient's reliability.

CONTROVERSY: Issues being debated regarding the management of preterm PROM include the use of steroids to accelerate pulmonary maturation, and antibiotic prophylaxis before the onset of labor. It is clear that as the days pass following PROM, the risk of chorioamnionitis increases. Therefore, some advocate induction of labor for those with ruptured membranes after 34 weeks or if adequate amounts of surfactant are present.

20
CHAPTER

Third Trimester Bleeding

Third trimester bleeding can result from something as trivial as a localized vaginal infection, or it can be the harbinger of hemorrhage and death. In the nonpregnant state, the uterus receives approximately 1% of cardiac output. In the third trimester, it receives 20% of an increased cardiac output. Uterine bleeding in the third trimester can be quite impressive. This chapter deals primarily with evaluation of the hemodynamically stable patient.

For those patients who arrive at the hospital literally pouring out blood, there are two immediate objectives of treatment: fluid replacement and delivery. Transfusions and fluid serve as a temporizing measure until delivery can be accomplished. Ultimately, the one sure way to stop severe obstetrical hemorrhage is to deliver the fetus and remove the placenta. Fortunately, patients rarely present with hemorrhage and hypovolemic shock. There are usually smaller bleeds that may serve as warnings.

EVALUATION OF A PATIENT WITH THIRD TRIMESTER BLEEDING

Third trimester bleeding occurs in approximately 4% of patients. This excludes those patients with bloody show—a physiologic event that is described later. About half will have an inconsequential cause, whereas the remainder will have either placenta previa or an abruption. Of course, those with a placenta previa who are bleeding are also frequently experiencing separation of the placenta from the uterine wall (abruption).

There are two diagnostic clues to discerning the cause of the bleeding: the history and the physical.

History

Ask about prior episodes, abdominal pain, uterine contractions, and recent intercourse. It is also important to ask a patient if she has had an ultrasound exam during the pregnancy and, if so, when. Although patients usually are not told where their placenta is located, most will be advised if it is actually covering the cervix.

Examination

Assessment of uterine contractions and tenderness is critical. Electronic fetal monitoring should be initiated to detect potential compromise. Finally, a gentle speculum exam should be performed in an effort to distinguish cervical from uterine bleeding (often difficult). During visualization of the cervix, some assessment should be made of dilatation.

CONTROVERSY: *There is some debate about whether a speculum exam should be done before knowing the location of the placenta. Some argue that the speculum exam can be as traumatic as a digital exam. It is certainly reasonable to do the ultrasound exam first if the situation permits.*

A digital cervical exam should not be done unless the placental location has been established by ultrasound. Prior to the widespread use of this test, it was common to examine patients with third trimester bleeding with the *double set-up examination.* This procedure entailed an exam in the cesarean section room with the patient prepped for an immediate cesarean section in case the examiner disrupted placental integrity in those with placenta previa. With the high accuracy of ultrasound, this is now rarely necessary.

Other Tests

As has already been mentioned, if an ultrasound has not identified the location of the placenta, one should be obtained. The prenatal Pap smear should be double-checked. As part of the evaluation, a CBC should be obtained, along with a coagulation profile (PT, PTT, D-dimer assay, and platelet count). For any patient who seems to have uterine bleeding, some blood should be cross-matched. The number of units that should be standing by depends on the circumstances, but 4 U is often a good place to start.

DIFFERENTIAL DIAGNOSIS

1. **Contact bleeding.** Because the cervix is more vascular during pregnancy, intercourse can rup-

ture a cervical blood vessel, resulting in bleeding that can be impressive. A recent pelvic exam to assess cervical dilatation also can be a source of this bleeding. This diagnosis is made when suggested by the history and when other causes are excluded.

2. **Cervical inflammation.** Occasionally, vaginal infections will cause the cervix to spontaneously bleed, although the quantity of blood is usually small. Again, other causes should be excluded.

3. **Cervical effacement and dilatation.** Occasionally, vaginal bleeding may be the presenting complaint of someone experiencing labor. Usually, bleeding during labor will be accompanied by the passage of cervical mucus, although this is not always the case. Rarely, the bleeding may be brisk enough to suggest other causes.

4. **Placenta previa.** This refers to the placenta preceding the fetus and actually covering the cervix. See the next section.

5. **Placental abruption.** Premature separation of the placenta from the uterine wall is known as abruption. This is discussed in a later section.

6. **Bloody show.** Bloody show is painless vaginal bleeding that is typically small to moderate in amount and occurs close to term. It can occur randomly and without obvious cause. Typically, although not always, it contains much mucus. It is so common that it may be regarded as a physiologic event, although it remains a diagnosis of exclusion.

7. **Other disorders.** Coagulation disorders and cervical cancer are very uncommon causes of third trimester bleeding. The initial labs should help suggest a coagulation disorder if one exists. Checking the prenatal Pap smear and visualizing the cervix can usually eliminate cancer as a cause.

PLACENTA PREVIA

Prior to the past century, placenta previa had roughly a 30% maternal mortality rate and was almost universally fatal for the fetus.

Incidence

Placenta previa occurs roughly once in every 250 pregnancies. Its incidence increases significantly as parity rises. **PEARL: Although a low-lying placenta may be visualized relatively frequently in the second trimester, in 90% of patients the condition resolves and does not pose problems as the uterus grows.** Placenta previa is somewhat more common in those who have had multiple abortions. The risk of recurrence in subsequent pregnancies is about 4% to 8%.

Diagnosis

The characteristic presentation of placenta previa is painless vaginal bleeding in the late second trimester or in the third trimester. The first episode of bleeding is most common near 34 weeks' gestation. Sometimes, placenta previa is associated with either an abruption or labor. The presence of contractions does not exclude this diagnosis.

There are several definitions of placenta previa worth reviewing. **PEARL: A *complete previa* means that the placenta is entirely covering the cervix. With a *partial previa,* the placenta covers only part of the cervical os. In a *marginal previa,* the placenta just reaches the cervix. Finally, a *low-lying placenta* is one near the cervical opening (common usage is within 2 cm) but not abutting it.**

This terminology obscures two important general principles. First, due to the changing anatomical relationship of the placenta to the uterus as the pregnancy progresses, most placentas that appear on ultrasound exam to be covering the cervix in early pregnancy are seen to move away from the cervix as the pregnancy progresses. **PEARL: If the placenta is not covering the cervix in early pregnancy, it will not move downward subsequently.** Therefore, it is usually unnecessary to repeat an ultrasound exam for placenta localization if a placenta is reported to be low lying in the first or second trimesters. Second, significant bleeding almost never occurs from placentas that are merely low lying. However, women in whom the placenta is actually seen to be covering all or a portion of the cervix require special management.

Treatment

Treatment consists of two approaches: delivery by cesarean and delay of delivery for as long as possible.

CONTROVERSY: The longer the pregnancy continues, the higher the risk of major hemorrhage. As a result, it is common practice to perform an amniocentesis for fetal lung maturity determination at 36 weeks. Fetuses with a low probability of respiratory distress syndrome are then promptly delivered.

Most patients with placenta previa will have repetitive episodes of bleeding. As a result, once the diagnosis of placenta previa is made, the patients are kept at bed rest for the remainder of the pregnancy, often in the hospital. For those patients hospitalized with frequent bouts of bleeding, it is common to have 2 to 4 U of blood typed and cross-matched at all times. Sometimes a large-bore IV line is maintained continuously until delivery.

The chief method of buying time for the fetus other than bed rest is through maternal blood transfusions. Again, because bleeding tends to be recurrent and unpredictable, most physicians try to keep the maternal hemoglobin above some arbitrary value to ensure adequate oxygenation for the fetus and some protection of the mother in the event of future blood loss.

CONTROVERSY: *Transfusing to keep the hemoglobin at 10 g or above is the figure most often cited in the literature.*

When bleeding episodes do occur in the hospital, it is wise to transfer the mother from the antepartum floor to labor and delivery for fetal monitoring and close observation. For anything but the most insignificant bleeding, preparations should be made for cesarean section. Patients with placenta previa may have to be moved to and from labor and delivery several times during the pregnancy.

Even with the strategy of bed rest in the hospital, blood transfusions, and cesarean birth, a good outcome cannot be guaranteed. The maternal mortality rate with this condition is at least somewhat increased, although it is less than 1%. The perinatal mortality rate is higher, on the order of 10% to 15%.

Complications

Several adverse outcomes are associated with placenta previa. Intrauterine growth retardation is thought to be more common, and the incidence of congenital anomalies is roughly doubled. One particularly fearsome complication is that of placenta accreta—a condition in which the placenta has abnormally attached to the myometrium. The result is that there is no smooth cleavage plane, and it is impossible to separate the placenta entirely from the uterine wall. As a result, the placental site continues to bleed following delivery. Often, the only cure for this problem is removal of the uterus, because less drastic measures seldom succeed in achieving hemostasis. Placenta accreta is a particular concern if the placenta previa occurs in a patient with a prior cesarean, but it can also occur with a normally located placenta. Placenta accreta poses a special problem because of the frequent difficulty in stopping bleeding without performing a hysterectomy. Such a hysterectomy performed in the immediate postpartum period is inherently difficult and prone to complications, particularly large blood loss.

ABRUPTION

Abruption refers to premature separation of the placenta from the uterine wall. This separation can be partial or complete. A clinically evident abruption poses a risk to both mother and fetus.

Incidence

Abruption is thought to complicate roughly 1% of all pregnancies. Hypertension, cigarette smoking, and even trauma (severe) all predispose the mother to placental separation. Those who have had a prior abruption are at increased risk for recurrence (roughly 6%). Abruption accounts for approximately 10% to 15% of all perinatal deaths. The risk to the fetus comes from anoxia, exsanguination, or premature delivery.

Diagnosis

The diagnosis of abruption is dependent on the history and physical. Ultrasound and lab studies can suggest the diagnosis, but the patient's presentation is key. **PEARL: The classic signs and symptoms of abruption are vaginal bleeding, uterine tenderness, and contractions.** Of course, in early or mild cases, some patients have only one of these problems at the outset.

Ultrasound is useful for excluding placenta previa but cannot reliably confirm the diagnosis of placental separation. A drop in hemoglobin or a decrease in coagulability also suggests the diagnosis, but again, it is the patient's signs and symptoms that are the key. **PEARL: Disseminated intravascular coagulation (DIC) occurs in less than 10% of cases and is more common in those with fetal demise or excessive blood loss.**

Management

PEARL: As with all cases of third trimester bleeding, establish first that the mother with abruption is hemodynamically stable by noting her pulse, blood pressure, skin color, mentation, and the like. Then establish heart tones and begin electronic fetal monitoring. Volume replacement, transfusion, and immediate delivery (by cesarean) are appropriate for mothers with continued bleeding, or for fetal distress. **PEARL: If the abruption is mild, the mother is stable, and there is no evidence of fetal distress, bed rest and observation, and even vaginal delivery for those in labor may be appropriate.**

DIC is one of the most serious complications of an abruption. DIC is characterized by spontaneous bleeding from places such as the nose or the IV site. Although the treatment of this complication is beyond the scope of this book, the approach usually consists of massive blood transfusions, immediate delivery, and occasionally, the use of a MAST suit. Once the fetus and placenta are delivered, the illness usually resolves spontaneously, although patients can become quite ill in the meantime.

21
CHAPTER

Forceps Delivery and Vacuum Extraction

The original use for forceps was to extract a dead baby from its mother. This situation was a desperate one, because safe cesarean section has only been available for the past century. Failure to extract the fetus would mean almost certain maternal death. Of course, for the past several centuries, forceps have been more commonly used to assist with difficult births. At present, forceps are used to shorten labor whenever the mother or fetus might benefit. They are no longer used when a difficult birth is anticipated, because most obstetricians resort to abdominal delivery in these circumstances.

DEFINITIONS

The definitions presented in the next section are taken from an American College of Obstetricians and Gynecologists Technical Bulletin of August 1994 and remain in current use. The cervix has to be completely dilated before forceps can be applied.

Outlet Forceps

Some conditions must be fulfilled for a delivery to qualify as outlet forceps. First, the sagittal suture has to be in the anteroposterior plane. This means that the fetus is within 45° of either direct occiput anterior or direct occiput posterior. **PEARL: Second, the scalp must be visible without separating the labia.** With these criteria, application of forceps qualifies as outlet forceps.

Low Forceps

Low forceps delivery entails the use of forceps when the leading part of the fetal skull is at station +2 cm or more. By definition, low forceps delivery can involve rotation of more than 45°.

Midforceps

A midforceps delivery describes application of the forceps when the fetal skull is above +2 cm station.

High Forceps

High forceps delivery is no longer done under any circumstances; this refers to the delivery of the unengaged fetus (above 0 station) by forceps.

INDICATIONS

The indications for forceps delivery involve the need to shorten labor to benefit either the mother or the fetus. One of the more common reasons for using forceps is maternal exhaustion.

CONTROVERSY: The American College of Obstetricians and Gynecologists suggests considering intervention in a nulliparous patient in the second stage after 3 hours with an epidural or after 2 hours without one. For a parous patient, the corresponding times are 2 hours and 1 hour, although these recommendations are somewhat arbitrary.

With electronic fetal monitoring, obstetricians are less compelled to deliver the fetus after some arbitrary length of time has elapsed than they might have been previously. Other circumstances include fetal distress or maternal heart disease.

CONTROVERSY: There is debate over the safety of midforceps deliveries, particularly those requiring significant rotation. Some information published in the medical literature suggests an increased morbidity rate for fetuses delivered by this technique. Because a meaningful prospective randomized trial would be impossible to conduct, the issue may never be resolved. Some of the information comes from deliveries that occurred 20 years ago or more, and it is particularly difficult to apply those experiences to current practice. Several decades ago, it was routine to deliver mothers by forceps from relatively high stations while they were given general anesthesia. Because this type of intervention was much more aggressive than current practice, data from this experience simply do not reflect more recent outcomes accurately. Nothing suggests any increased morbidity from delivery using low or outlet forceps.

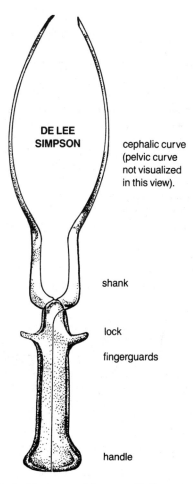

Figure 21–1. Features of forceps (DeLee modification of Simpson forceps). Note that the pelvic curve is not visualized in this view. (Adapted from Dennen, PC: Dennen's Forceps Deliveries, ed 3. FA Davis, Philadelphia, 1989, p 18, with permission.)

TECHNIQUE

Before applying forceps, the patient's bladder should be emptied and the fetal position confirmed. A pudendal block provides some benefit, but regional anesthesia is often preferable. **PEARL: After a forceps delivery, a special effort should be made to inspect the vaginal walls for lacerations, particularly near the ischial spines.** Occasionally, the delivery may prove to be more difficult than anticipated, in which case a cesarean section may be performed.

The forceps themselves can be described by four features (Fig. 21–1). The **blade** is the portion that actually grasps the fetus. Its **cephalic curve** corresponds to the shape of the fetal head, and the **pelvic curve** conforms to the general architecture of the maternal pelvis. Blades can be solid or hollowed out for a more firm application. The second feature of forceps is the **shank,** which connects the blade to the lock and handle. The shanks can

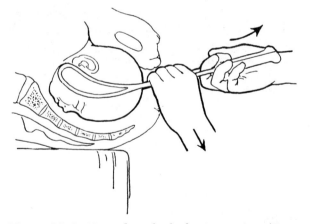

Figure 21–2. Manual method of axis traction. (From Dennen, PC: Dennen's Forceps Deliveries, ed 3. FA Davis, Philadelphia, 1989, p 57, with permission.)

either overlap or be separate. The **lock** is the portion that actually holds the two branches together. Finally, the **handle** is the part that is grasped by the obstetrician.

The method of application depends on the forceps and the position of the fetus. In general, the blades are designed for application to the sides of the fetal head rather than from front to back. It is often helpful to apply traction during a contraction, while having the mother push at the same time (Fig. 21–2). With low forceps or midforceps, the delivery often takes several contractions to accomplish.

VACUUM EXTRACTION

The principles for forceps delivery also apply to vacuum extraction. With this technique, a cup is placed on the fetal scalp and suction is applied to create an airtight seal. Either an electric or hand-powered pump may provide the suction. **PEARL: When using the vacuum, care must be taken to be sure that maternal tissues are not included in the application.** With the hand-powered vacuum devices commonly used today, the seal is readily broken if too much force is applied. In comparison to forceps, the vacuum extractor provides less traction but also less chance of vaginal lacerations.

Epilogue

At the time of this third edition, I have been in private practice for 12 years. These years have provided me with an interesting perspective on my residency experience and career choice.

I went into obstetrics and gynecology for four main reasons. This surgical specialty offers an opportunity for decisive intervention and cure. It also focuses heavily on preventive medicine in terms of contraception, sexually transmitted disease detection and prevention, and prenatal care. By and large, the delivery of babies is a very happy experience. Perhaps the most important reason for choosing this specialty is the ability to establish long-term contact with individual patients. Although much of medicine becomes routine and dull given enough time, the "normal vaginal birth in bed 120B" has more meaning if it is Mrs. Smith whom I have known for several years.

Malpractice crisis and increased government interference notwithstanding, I have found the four reasons given earlier to be largely valid. Although I am not particularly good at remembering names and faces, I find it particularly satisfying when I can link a name on the phone or the appointment list with someone I know. This is not often achievable in a residency program, where contact with a particular patient is limited by the length of a rotation.

I do not like getting out of bed in the middle of the night any more than the next person, but I still get a thrill out of deliveries. There is something marvelous about witnessing the first moments of a new life. Perhaps it will help medical students and junior residents to know that, at least for me, the struggle was worth it.

A
APPENDIX

Commonly Used Abbreviations

AFP.	Alpha-fetoprotein
AROM.	Artificial rupture of membranes
BPD.	Biparietal diameter
BPM.	Beats per minute
CPD.	Cephalopelvic disproportion
EDC.	Estimated date of confinement
FHR.	Fetal heart rate
FHT.	Fetal heart tones
HPI.	History of present illness
IUFD.	Intrauterine fetal demise
IUGR.	Intrauterine growth retardation
IUPC.	Intrauterine pressure catheter
LMP.	Last menstrual period
LTV.	Long-term variability
NST.	Nonstress test
NTD.	Neural tube defect
PIH.	Pregnancy-induced hypertension
PMH.	Past medical history
PROM.	Premature rupture of membranes
ROS.	Review of systems
SROM.	Spontaneous rupture of membranes
STV.	Short-term variability
VBAC.	Vaginal birth after cesarean

Index